Praise for Shakesp

"*Shakespeare's Yoga* gives the reader a new way of looking at the plays of Shakespeare, which is quite an accomplishment on the 400th anniversary of his legacy! This book represents a truly unique blend of the Bard and yogic wisdom. It will be of great interest to lovers of Shakespeare and devotees of yoga."

—Laura Bates, author of *Shakespeare Saved My Life: Ten Years in Solitary with the Bard*

"A beautiful narrative of faith, timelessness, and the depth of living. Two great forces of spirituality, Shakespeare and Patanjali, are united in opening a new dialog to living with our complex, kindest, truest version of ourselves."

—Will Duprey, author of *Form: A Poetic Experience of the Hatha Yoga Pardipika*

"Whether you have yet to experience yoga or Shakespeare—or are an expert in either or both—*Shakespeare's Yoga* takes you into a profound and valuable exploration of life's big questions. Claire Szabo-Cassella has pulled together yogic philosophy, excerpts from Shakespeare's work, and an array of quotations and inspiration from those invested on the path of yoga as well as those immersed in the world of Shakespeare to create a life-affirming companion to your journey on and off the mat."

—Heidi E. Spear, MA, author, Kripalu yoga teacher, meditation coach, and a creator of the workshop The Yoga of Shakespeare

"Warmly and wisely written, *Shakespeare's Yoga* savors the Bard's timelessness and how it can deepen our inner embodiment of the yoga experience. A rare and transformative read for yogis and Shakespeare lovers alike."

—Sarahjoy Marsh, MA, yoga teacher, yoga therapist
and author of *Hunger, Hope, and Healing*

"*Shakespeare's Yoga* is a unique contribution to yoga literature. Claire Szabo-Cassella's insights on Shakespeare and Patanjali shed new light on the path of yoga and will help deepen your practice."

—Colin Clements, publisher of *Australia Yoga Life*

"Creatively deep and unique. *Shakespeare's Yoga* will provide anyone with a love for yoga and Shakespeare a page-turning experience. This book is blending the wisdom of the ages with modern-day interpretations. Wonderful, complex, and an important literary work!"

—HawaH, founder and editor of *The Poetry of Yoga* anthology

Shakespeare's Yoga

Shakespeare's Yoga

How the Bard Can Deepen Your Practice—On and Off the Mat

CLAIRE SZABO-CASSELLA

White Cloud Press
Ashland, Oregon

All rights reserved. Copyright © 2016 by Claire Szabo-Cassella.
No part of this book may be reproduced or transmitted in any form or
by any means whatsoever, including graphic, electronic, or mechanical,
including photocopying, recording, taping, or by any information storage
or retrieval system, without permission from the publisher.

White Cloud Press titles may be purchased for educational, business, or sales
promotional use. For information, please write: Special Market Department,
White Cloud Press, PO Box 3400, Ashland, OR 97520
Website: www.whitecloudpress.com

Cover and Interior Design by Christy Collins, C Book Services

First edition: 2016
16 17 18 19 20   10 9 8 7 6 5 4 3 2 1

Library of Congress Cataloging-in-Publication Data

Names: Szabo-Cassella, Claire, author.
Title: Shakespeare's yoga : how the bard can deepen your practice--on and off
  the mat / Claire Szabo-Cassella.
Description: Ashland, OR : White Cloud Press, 2016.
Identifiers: LCCN 2016007763 | ISBN 9781940468389 (paperback)
Subjects: LCSH: Hatha yoga. | BISAC: HEALTH & FITNESS / Yoga.
Classification: LCC RA781.7 .S95 2016 | DDC 613.7/046--dc23
LC record available at http://lccn.loc.gov/2016007763

MIX
Paper from
responsible sources
FSC
www.fsc.org   FSC® C011935

To Shakespeare and Patanjali for lighting the path,
and to my loving husband, Lou, for sharing the journey

Table of Contents

Acknowledgments

Writing a first book is a lesson in gratitude. I am evermore thankful to Professor James "Doc" Ayres for instilling the joy of self-discovery that comes with exploring Shakespeare's words on stage; Professor William B. Worthen for furthering my academic study of Shakespeare off stage; Professor Laura Bates for her wise guidance throughout the writing process of this book; David Ziegler for his friendship and continual support; Dennis Skipper for his astute and thorough edits; Casey Palmer and the *sangha* of Near East Yoga for their dynamic study of the *Yoga Sutras*; Richard Heinzkill for championing my study of all things Shakespeare; David Sabo for his financial generosity; Steve Scholl for his warm welcome, diplomacy and care as my publisher; my parents for investing so selflessly in my liberal arts education; and, to my touchstone, a source of unending love and creative support, my husband Lou Cassella.

Introduction

Was Shakespeare "enlightened"?

That is the question a growing number of yogis and authors on spirituality are answering with a resounding "Ay!" (That's "yes" in Elizabethan lingo).

Sure, the Bard probably never sat bound in Lotus Position (*padmasana*)—that could be challenging if one is sporting a doublet, I imagine—nor did he likely lead a "yogic" lifestyle enmeshed in the Elizabethan theater world. Still, his plays illuminate the beauty and purpose of our human condition with an uncommon clarity. This was a playwright who was awake and aware of the true nature of "reality," the dream-like state of our existence, and the roles we play in acting out our personal dramas like costumed actors on a stage or in a yoga studio. With an ever-changing timeliness, Shakespeare's plays bear witness to our own stories and do so with the powerful ability to elevate and transform the meaning of our practice and our existence. Our ethical potential is reflected in his characters, both comically and tragically. Learning from their choices equips us better for life itself. As a result, audiences continue to applaud Shakespeare for an honest, good look at what our ego and divine selves are capable of that, hopefully, helps us to make better-informed choices between the two—on and off the mat. Only an "enlightened master" can inspire such penetrating wisdom for 400 years and counting.

The more I practice yoga, the more I appreciate Shakespeare. After twenty years on the mat as a yoga student, teacher, trainer, and cofounder of three studios, I better understand the Shakespearean lines I once played onstage at a theater called

Shakespeare at Winedale (Texas). While I studied the *Yoga Sutras* (a series of 196 aphorisms—small but mighty bits of yogic teaching—written in Sanskrit about 2000 years ago), my thoughts kept repeating, *Hey, Shakespeare said something remarkably similar! And in English! And with a humor and pathos that still leave me begging for more* (the yogic principle of nonattachment, *vairagya*, notwithstanding).

Thanks to my yoga practice I better comprehend the crucial importance of Shakespeare's core themes and spiritual wisdom, especially his recurring reminder on the integrity of Self. In *Hamlet*, Polonius counsels his college-bound son Laertes, "This above all: to thine own self be true" (*Hamlet* 1.3). Laertes's dad is usually played as a self-absorbed, shallow fool and this fatherly advice viewed as a platitudinous invitation to do whatever makes Laertes feel good (Bill Murray's portrayal in the 2000 film version being a notable exception). To a yogi, however, realizing the critical interplay between the illusion of a truly separate self and the true Self—the *atman*, soul, or divine nature—takes a lifetime (maybe thousands of them). This directive is the basis of yoga philosophy, including yoga psychotherapist Stephen Cope's book entitled *Yoga and the Quest for the True Self*. Each Shakespearean play, like every yoga practice, is an open-ended opportunity to encounter the story of our life as just a play unfolding. The ego-directed self, with its panache for theatricality and drama, makes being true to the higher Self noble work, just the opposite of self-serving. Because when we're true to who we really are, we act with a heightened awareness of our every thought, word, and action and their effects on our lives and others, including animals and the planet. It's what the journey is "above all" all about—our interconnectedness.

When viewed through the yogic lens, Polonius's oft-quoted advice certainly gives us another way of looking at what he is suggesting and to whom; his words are not just for his son's journey, but for ours too. He, like many of Shakespeare's "fools," is a superb yoga teacher in disguise. Polonius is ultimately advising that one achieve a balance—a basic reason for practicing yoga—and be a responsible and self-realized person.

Of course many other great modern authors have also touched on the universal themes of living a well-examined life, but Shakespeare's inventive use of language got to our hearts and imaginations first. How his voice captures the inner dynamics of characters ranging from drunkards to magicians to kings, villains, and lovers (sometimes all within the same play!) with such an egoless accuracy remains a mystery explained only by inspiration (which translates as the breath of divine influence), not unlike the enigmatic origins of yoga itself.

Entertainment versus enter-train-ment

Shakespeare and yoga both offer benefits to even the absolute beginner on the very first encounter. Our bodies and minds are hardwired to benefit from all forms of yoga: conscious movement (*asana*), breathing exercises (*pranayama*), and the self-improvement that comes from exploring the human experience from a spiritual perspective (*svadhyaya*). And, as with Hamlet (a yoga philosopher in the extreme), asking ourselves the big questions—Who's there? What if? Who am I? What am I? To be or not to be?—comes naturally when given the inspiration, time, and space to do so. These same inquiries and more arise during our yoga practice: Who is breathing me? Where does the energy moving my body come from? Where do the images in my mind come from and go to? If Hamlet were in our yoga class, the only difference between him and us would be that he'd be speaking his thoughts aloud, a theatrical device Shakespeare made famous, called soliloquy.

It is the answers to those questions that Shakespeare's enlightened insights radically shift within us, raising our consciousness and our ability to heal ourselves—and our world. That is how *any* form of yoga, including Shakespeare's yoga, works best: by mobilizing philosophy into right action. As the playwright, Shakespeare puts that job in our court. He is like a life coach who, also like a good yoga teacher, leaves the perception of his teachings on the human condition ultimately up to us.

But education without direct application has little value. Shakespeare's works and our local yoga classes are merely entertainment unless we choose to make the teachings "enter-train-ment" instead. The inherent guidance found within the plays and our yoga practice exists to lessen our struggles and direct our sails toward calmer, saner, and healthier lives—if we follow the advice given.

What we do after our revels are ended, once the stage clears and we roll up our mats, can transform what would be merely a physical and mental "exercise" into a catalyst for positive change in our lives. Given the opportunity to begin again, what can we do better, moving forward? Can we pause and recall Shakespeare's powerful examples of the importance of compassion (*karuna*, a form of *ahimsa*, or nonviolence), honesty (*satya*), faith (*shraddha*), contentment (*santosha*), surrender (*Ishvara pranidhana*), illusion (*maya*) and many other principles of yoga before we react? "Ay, there's the rub!" (*Hamlet* 3.1), as Shakespeare writes.

But I'm not flexible

There are many common fallacies about yoga and about Shakespeare. Despite popular notions, yoga is about so much more than touching your toes; and Shakespeare is not a club for the intellectually elite or white folks with money. Inspiring books and documentaries on the use of both Shakespeare and yoga in prisons, refugee camps, and the schools of disadvantaged youth have proved to be positive, often life-changing endeavors for everyone involved: teachers, students, actors, directors, audiences, and communities. These are arts that do more than just temporarily relieve the suffering of our predicament or diseases; they offer experiential wisdom that improves self-esteem, confidence, and communication skills—including how we relate to our self, first and foremost.

Anyone committed to these experiences undergoes a sea change, an internal shift that illuminates the truth of who they really are and what they're capable of as essentially loving beings. These processes require taking an honest good look at our character as multifaceted and pliable. Do we recognize that what we watch or perform onstage is a potential part of own character? Does our yoga practice in daily life reflect the truth of our spirit? Can we accept our contradictory nature and embrace the whole of life? Participating in a Shakespearean play and participating in a yoga class couldn't be more similar. They teach us the awesome power and responsibility we possess to become more self-aware.

The practice never ends

Yoga, like unpeeling the layers of meaning in Shakespeare, is an infinite game, a practice that never ends. In the 2012 documentary *Shakespeare High*, Richard Dreyfuss talks about the complex nature of Shakespeare: "You've got to work immediately just to understand it and what he is saying . . . . And just when you start to unpeel the lessons offered, you find the gesture never ends."[1] His comments beg the question: Has this Academy Award–winning actor also practiced yoga? These same remarks could easily be found in many yoga books.

---

1. *Shakespeare High*, DVD, directed by Alex Rotaru, (New York: Cinema Guild, 2012).

In the midst of an especially challenging posture, I smile while reminding my yin yoga students, "It's *just* yoga. And *anything* is only as hard or enjoyable as you imagine it to be, even Dragon Pose (a deep runner's lunge); just ask Shakespeare: 'There is nothing either good or bad but thinking makes it so' (*Hamlet* 2.2)." A snicker of laughter is a good sign that a student has shifted from an expectation of an immediate result to enjoying a cumulative process that is not expected to be easy or reach an end goal any time soon.

In a *Shakespeare Uncovered* episode, when commenting on playing Macbeth, screen legend Orson Wells sums up encountering Shakespeare by saying, "It is a great feeling to be dealing with material which is better than yourself, that you know you can never live up to."[2] Awe is as good for a Shakespearean actor as it is for any yogi. To redefine our participation as play rather than work makes an invaluable difference. A little humility and sense of perspective goes a long way, too.

Despite its unfathomable depth of experience, we all live with a body and mind that can benefit from some yoga—in this case, Shakespeare's take on the practice. Simply show up and open up to what you can do and what it means for you today, right now. Be advised, however: Shakespeare and yoga are not passive practices; they are potent arts. Presence and participation makes the magic work. Do what you can. Repeat, and expect positive results. With steady and consistent repetitions, the understanding and practice of both Shakespeare and yoga gets easier (at least somewhat), more interesting, and more fun. ("Fun" is not a typo.) More happiness is a natural by-product of any wisdom practice designed to last a lifetime.

---

2. *Shakespeare Uncovered: Macbeth with Ethan Hawke*, DVD, directed by Nicola Stockley (London: Blakeway Productions, 2012).

Practicing Shakespeare's yoga—on and off the mat

This book is a companion for your journey. It offers helpful suggestions for applying some of the Bard's most famous quotes and passages to your understanding of conscious living. In the chapters ahead, if certain themes touch an aspect of your life, seek out the whole play via live theater, movies, or a copy of the text when and where you can. Find a theater class that includes Shakespeare. Be curious and bold.

Likewise, if you've been wondering what the yoga buzz is all about, well, you've just found a very powerful—and healing—form of yoga in which to start your practice: the study of "sacred texts" (another definition of svadhyaya), among which Shakespeare's works are often considered to be included (no mat or spandex clothing required).

If you practice yoga already, knowledge of Shakespeare will enable you to make interesting connections to your practice on the mat and in daily life. The Bard presents characters akin to Arjuna in the Bhagavad Gita and plots echoing the philosophy of the Upanishads and contemporary metaphysics. The focus of our comparison, however, is on the ethical guidelines found in Patanjali's *Yoga Sutras*, specifically the first limb of the Eight-Limb Path, called the *yamas* (more on that in just a bit). From there, we can turn the play inward, hold the mirror up to our nature, and witness how we, like Shakespeare's characters, can better juggle our virtues with our vices at every stage of our practice.

This book is relevant to anyone wanting to deepen a lifetime practice of self-growth with yogic insights from the literary master on the human condition. Yoga students of every level, shape, and size, as well as Shakespearean actors, theatergoers, and instructors, can use this book to find renewal and fresh ideas. As a result, application of Shakespeare's yogic teachings changes your life and how you view it, as that is the inherent promise of yoga itself—personal transformation.

It has mine.

The two gentlemen of yoga: Patanjali and Shakespeare

Moving forward, it will be helpful to know more about the Bard and the person some revere as the father of yoga, Patanjali. There are striking similarities between these two collectors and dispensers of ancient wisdom.

To begin, we don't really know much about either one of them.

Shakespeare's life and authorship have been the source of unending debate. He was born a commoner in Stratford-upon-Avon, England, on April 23, 1564, and died on exactly the same date fifty-two years later. (Yes, I find that coincidence rather remarkable, too.) A few public tax records and questionable portraits bear his name and likeness, but that's it. If literary historians unearth even a smidgen of a morsel of new information, believe me, it makes the headlines.

Patanjali lived in what is now called India, somewhere around 200 BCE to 400 CE. He could be one of several different scholars around that time, the incarnation of Adisesa (a mythical serpent), or maybe a woman (I have heard a yoga lecturer refer to Patanjali-a for that very possibility!). It bears noting that there is also very little concrete evidence on the personal lives of other great spiritual teachers. Jesus, Buddha, Muhammad, and Lao-Tzu all have as brief and contested biographies as have Shakespeare and Patanjali.

The point is this: don't go there. They existed—in some form. They both drew from the sources they knew intimately (somehow) and re-presented ethical philosophies designed to help us better understand who *we* are and what we think *we're* doing here.

Second, both the Bard and Patanjali were artistic entrepreneurs of sorts.

Shakespeare borrowed ideas, generously, from Montaigne, Plato, Ovid, Holinshed's Chronicles (history books of the day), and his local competitors. However, he made similar plots and characters supremely richer by his choice of words, making up a couple thousand new words as he scratched out 38 plays[3] and 154 sonnets with a quill and ink. No writer has come remotely close to the number of words Shakespeare added to the English language. This was an author who knew how to use creative license to render emotion very, very well.

Traditionally, Patanjali is credited with writing the *Yoga Sutras*. As mentioned earlier, this is a compilation of 196 threads—or sutras—of wisdom divided over four books (*padas*). These brief, interchangeable lessons on yoga encapsulate the best of all prior ancient wisdom, including the Vedas and the Upanishads (more on the *Yoga Sutras* in just a bit too).

Next, both authors refrain from trying to control our behavior. They guide it.

Shakespeare and Patanjali understood that the human experience involves making constant choices, planting seeds of cause and effect, each of which holds a consequence (karma). Both authors serve as our guides, spiritual teachers who understand the important interplay between darkness (ignorance) and light (true wisdom). Through their books and plays, they impart enlightened wisdom that encourages us to plant good seeds to avoid future suffering.

As the author of *Shakespeare's Wife*, Germaine Greer comments in a *Shakespeare Uncovered* episode, "One of the important things about Shakespeare is he's not trying to *say* anything; he's not trying

---

3.   Make that 39 plays if you include the recent discovery of Shakespeare's reported lost play, *Cardenio*.

to tell you how to think, what he is saying is: *think*."[4] Likewise, Patanjali illuminates the path to a calmer mind and a healthier, happier existence, but he doesn't dictate a better or worse way to get on that path or which direction is best for whom. The journey is the path. The play is the practice. The guru of the theater and the yogic sage present the same truths on the art of right living. They ask us to take a look at our mental, emotional, and physical patterns (*samskaras*) and create ourselves anew rather than be fortune's fool. Each pivotal moment is up to us.

Finally, both of their works are designed to be lived, not just read—by everyone.

Shakespeare never saw his plays in print. His colleagues John Heminges and Henry Condell pieced together the scripts and remembered scraps of actor dialogue into a collection of his plays, called the First Folio, in 1623, eight years after Shakespeare's death. (And what a debt of gratitude the world owes them for their efforts.) Shakespeare wrote for live theater—a messy, noisy, very lively place of transformational words and movements. He was a social-media magnate in his day. Besides gossip, theater is where average people turned to for news. Political, religious, and social events of the day were explored onstage (obliquely, as what was often reflected onstage was the offstage political debate of some mighty powerful patronage: Queen Elizabeth until 1603 and then King James I). Unless the plague was rampant or a monarchy change underway, people packed the theater seven days a week to learn more about their world and themselves. People just like you and me.

When Shakespeare died, his notable contemporary Ben Jonson was—and still is—often quoted as eulogizing, "He was not of an age, but for all time." Some 400 years later, Jonson's observation

---

4. *Shakespeare Uncovered: The Comedies: Twelfth Night and As You Like It with Joely Richardson*, DVD, directed by Janice Sutherland (London: Blakeway Productions, 2012). Emphasis added.

holds true. Shakespeare's plays are now as popular in Japan as they are in his homeland; his lines, even when misquoted out of context, add weight to speakers' conversations; and the infinite variety of adaptations made of his plays can arise only because of their timeless universality.

On the importance of playing Shakespeare, cofounder of the Royal Shakespeare Company, John Barton, makes this point as a director: "The sort of points that need to be made [about how to act Shakespeare] could only arise, truly, in the context of working with actors. Each actor and his experience is worth many books. What I have to say is, in the end, it's worth nothing if it doesn't come alive in the performance of living and breathing actors."[5] As a yoga teacher, I couldn't agree more. Substitute Shakespeare's name with Patanjali's and the word "actor" with "student," and you describe the purpose of teaching yoga—to awaken people to their potential physically, emotionally, and spiritually.

Likewise, Patanjali's *Yoga Sutras* were originally chanted or sung. He never saw his verses in print. Some sects recited the sutras prior to meals, keeping the wisdom alive in periods of waning use (again, what a debt of gratitude the world owes them for their efforts). The *Yoga Sutras* are succinct verses, strung together like jewels on a string (hence the Sanskrit term *sutra* that means "string, thread") that enable wisdom to be passed down orally from teacher to student; notebooks and recorders were unimaginable and not necessary back in Patanjali's day. Student discipline and trust in the teacher's ability to translate the verse got the job done. Still today, chanting the sutras in their original and evocative Sanskrit adds to the power of their understanding while keeping the oral tradition of their teaching alive and well.

---

5. *Playing Shakespeare with the Royal Shakespeare Company*, TV Mini-Series, directed by John Carlaw and Peter Walker (London: London Weekend Television, 1982).

Patanjali poses the question: Why yoga? His answers are wise advice for daily living that we can chant, read, study, reference, and write about still today. The knowledge Patanjali passes down contains five universal truths (yamas):

○ **ahimsa:** nonviolence
○ **satya:** truthfulness
○ **asteya:** nonstealing
○ **brahmacharya:** moderation and balance, awareness of Divinity
○ **aparigraha:** nonpossessiveness

Elaborating on these yamas Patanjali says, "These universals, transcending birth, place, era or circumstance, constitute the great vow of yoga" (*Yoga Sutra* 2.31).[6]

This great vow is more than just a code of conduct; it constitutes a way of being that honors the mysterious interrelatedness of life despite cultural differences. But, to echo the Shakespearean director John Barton, they are worthless aphorisms unless they come alive in our practice of conscious living.

More and more people today show up at the yoga mat for a similar purpose—to quench a deep-seated curiosity about how we move, think, and exist as individuals sharing the communal experience of being human. The sage's insightful exploration into our human condition is as revered in yoga circles as are Shakespeare's texts in the literary world.

By recognizing Shakespeare plays as an enlightened source in which to further inspire and inform our practice, we find that "all the world's a stage" (*As You Like It* 2.7) for yoga practice. And we as actors play a leading role as yogis in evolving the world into a better place with each conscious breath and movement. Bringing

---

6. Chip Hartranft, trans., *The Yoga-Sutra of Patanjali* (Boston & London: Shambhala, 2003), 32.

Shakespeare and Patanjali together—on and off the mat—empowers our every effort.

More on the Yoga Sutras

Patanjali's *Yoga Sutras* offer serenity for the tempests of the mind and healing for the diseases of the body. In book two (*Sadhana Pada*) and book three (*Vibhuti Pada*), the sage details an Eight-Limb Path for enlightened living, called *ashtanga* (not to be confused with a popular yoga modality devised by the late Sri Pattabhi Jois, who died in 2009). If you follow the practices along this Eight-Limb Path, you will realize supernatural powers—better thought of as heightened sensitivities, or *siddhis*: a stronger intuition, greater serendipity, insights into the nature of life and your purpose for being here, just to name a few. Your life will change for the better. Trials and difficult emotions will still arise (guaranteed), but you'll have tools to handle them with greater ease and grace.

Although there are many different ways onto the path, if the path is followed, our struggles lessen and our happiness grows. As a framework for *Shakespeare's Yoga*, concentrating on the yamas is where our time and energy will be wisely spent. Regardless of time, condition, or class, we are purified and unified (with each other, ourselves, and all other sentient beings) by the yamas. Shakespeare's works are filled with these themes. And we will explore Shakespeare's parallel depiction of each yama one by one.

Before we dive into those chapters, however, I want to give you some context as to how the yamas relate to the other seven limbs, especially the *niyamas* (the second limb).

The Eight-Limb Path of Patanjali

1st Limb: **yamas**—external practices in our dealings with others, moral harmony

There are five yamas (which we explore in this book):

- ○ **ahimsa:** nonviolence
- ○ **satya:** truthfulness
- ○ **asteya:** nonstealing
- ○ **brahmacharya:** moderation and balance, awareness of Divinity
- ○ **aparigraha:** nonpossessiveness

2nd Limb: **niyamas**—personal observances in how we treat ourselves

There are five niyamas:

- ○ **saucha:** cleanliness
- ○ **santosha:** contentment
- ○ **tapas:** discipline
- ○ **svadhyaya:** self-study
- ○ **Isvara pranidhana:** surrender to the Divine

3rd Limb: **asana:** postures

4th Limb: **pranayama:** breath control, harnessing the life force

5th Limb: **pratyahara:** withdrawal of the senses

6th Limb: **dharana:** concentration

7th Limb: **dhyana:** meditation

8th Limb: **samadhi:** union with the Divine

Mission possible

The core teachings of the *Yoga Sutras*, including the eight precepts and their subteachings above, point us in the right direction—onto the path, one that leads to a greater awareness of what it means to be awake. Some suggest that the Eight-Limb Path unfolds sequentially, one precept leading naturally to the next, and to a large degree that is absolutely true. But, as is the case with most

Westerners who jump on the path via the postures (the 3rd limb—asana), being on one limb of the path will naturally involve participating in the other seven limbs. It's a package deal.

This same interconnectedness is especially true of the yamas and niyamas. In his book, *Light on the Yoga Sutras of Patanjali*, B.K.S. Iyengar writes:

> The observance of *yama* brings about *niyama*, and the practice of *niyama* disciplines one to follow the principles of *yama*. For example, nonviolence brings purity of thought and deed, truthfulness leads to contentment, and non-covetousness leads to tapas. Chastity leads to the study of the self, and non-possessiveness to surrender to God.[7]

The yamas are socially oriented, the essential principles for interacting well with others; the niyamas are more internally focused, principles describing how best to take charge of our own growth and well-being. In her book, *The Yamas & Niyamas*,[8] Deborah Adele sums up these two ethical philosophies with a provocative and humorous analogy, one she found on a mug:

Things to do today:
1. Stop the Arms Race
2. Floss

From large to small, the moment-to-moment thoughts, words, and actions we engage in throughout our daily existence make a difference in our world and in our way of life. As we serve the change we want to see in the world, we become it. Random acts of kindness make a positive impact. Our little light illuminates a world of darkness.

---

7. B. K. S. Iyengar, *Light on the Yoga Sutras of Patanjali* (London: Thorsons, 1993), 31.
8. Deborah Adele, *The Yamas & Niyamas: Exploring Yoga's Ethical Practice* (Duluth, Minnesota: On-Word Bound Books, 2009), 12.

Shakespeare and the great vow of yoga

Okay, back to basics: the yamas. And the task at hand: exploring Shakespeare's timeless examples of them.

The term *yamas* often translates as "self-restraints" or "yoga don'ts," probably because of literal takes on Sanskrit word construction and as an analogy to the strict and stern Ten Commandments perhaps necessary at the time of that translation. The first yama, *ahimsa*, for example, breaks down as *a* (meaning "opposite of" or "against") and *hims* (meaning "to strike or harm") or, when put together, "nonviolence." "Don't kill any living being," however, may not be as inspiring a translation as the social interactions that *act*-ualize ahimsa—words and behaviors such as compassion and forgiveness. For example, *asteya*, or "nonstealing," is best realized through honesty and generosity. For this reason, I periodically include the English translation of each yama. I also draw from both masculine and feminine interpretations of the yoga sutras from which the yamas are derived, in order to represent a well-rounded view of Shakespeare's same spiritual lesson.

Patanjali's yamas and Shakespeare's plays are not so much about "right or wrong" or who's the villain or the heroine, as such conclusions are often based on popular opinion and personal perception; rather, their works ask us to consider, deeply consider, our patterns of reaction to life's dramas, as these are the grains that will grow with time. When situations arise and we are faced with options in thought, word, or action, both sage and playwright have our highest destiny in mind—that of evolving our individual and collective consciousness back to our divine and unified origins.

Shakespeare's plays unite us because we feel a connection to the humanness of his characters' predicaments and their potential for grace. By recognizing that their dramas, which are illusionary and temporary states (maya), are alive and well in all of us regardless of time, race, or location, we unify over a glimpse of our universal morality and the importance of our personal dedication to "the great vow of yoga," the choiceless choices of right living better known as the yamas. The sage explains the universal principles of the yamas in Sanskrit; the playwright portrays his characters' use—or misuse—of the same absolute truths onstage. When applied or abused, the results are the same in both the imaginary world of the theater and in our lives: either more or less suffering, depending on how well one chooses the keys that open that spiritual gate and set us all free: compassion, truthfulness, generosity, balance and moderation, and gratitude—the positive connotations of the yamas.

Onward. The journey awaits. And, to quote an Elizabethan yoga teacher named Shakespeare:

> *We came into the world like brother and brother;*
> *And now let's go hand in hand, not one before another.*
> *—The Comedy of Errors* 5.1

Ahimsa

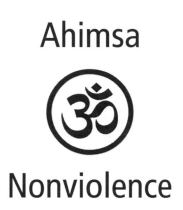

Nonviolence

CHAPTER 1
Ahimsa as Reflected
in *The Tempest*

The rarer action is
In virtue than in vengeance.
−*The Tempest* 5.1

Ahimsa (nonviolence) is the primary yama because of its foundational importance on the path to spiritual enlightenment. Whatever other yoga practices we engage in (including the remaining four yamas), they must include ahimsa or any benefits are negated. It's that essential. Ahimsa is also the wellspring of true strength and power.

> By sticking to the principles of non-violence, one acquires
> strength and power as well as friendliness. (*Yoga Sutra* 3.24)[1]

Shakespeare offers superb examples of ahimsa. His plays are brimming with themes of compassion, friendship, and forgiveness. They are also chock-full of lessons on how violence occurs, lessons that circle back to the necessity of practicing ahimsa—and what happens when a hero or we as yogis act otherwise.

Shakespeare's plays stimulate socio-emotional learning at its best. And theater directors, educators, and behavioral experts in nonviolence are taking note. They are turning to Shakespeare to raise awareness of the cyclical nature of violence, patterns that are readily recognizable in his plays.

---

1. B. K. S. Iyengar, trans., *Core of the Yoga Sutras: The Definitive Guide to the Philosophy of Yoga* (London: HarperThorsons, 2012), 145.

Dr. Beverly Kingston, director of the Center for the Study and Prevention of Violence (Colorado) looks to Shakespeare as an educational tool. She says, "Shakespeare's plays are tools that bring forth issues surrounding human violence. They are superb resources that teach relationship skills and the power of empathy. His plays also tell what not to do when these situations arise." As the CSPV director pointed out to me, "When there is an intent to harm; when a harmful act is repeated over time and escalates; and when a power imbalance is present, be aware. Violence is present but future violence is preventable."[2]

Yoga moments

Kingston's insights into violence prevention prove true in *The Tempest*, one of Shakespeare's last plays. In the wake of a rude and noisy storm, characters address matters of personal freedom and forgiveness, issues that have been brewing for twelve years. It's a plotline headed for unpleasant, if not tragic, results until Prospero, a royal alchemist out for revenge, gets a grip on what constitutes true nobility, true magic: ahimsa. It takes him all five acts of the play, but he gets there. By uncoloring his disturbed mind (*aklishta*), he consciously chooses to pardon his politically ambitious brother, Antonio, who successfully plotted to usurp his kingdom and left him and his baby daughter islanded somewhere between Milan and Tunis (that's in Africa, not Italy). Interpretations vary as to whether Prospero's plan is calculated retaliation or harmless restitution. In both scenarios, however, his anger and magical mayhem escalate throughout the play until his dear, delicate Ariel, a spirit, teaches him a little yoga—a lesson in compassion.

---

2.   Dr. Beverly Kingston, interview with author, 18 June 2014.

ARIEL
Your charm so strongly works 'em
That if you now beheld them, your affections
Would become tender.

PROSPERO
Dost thou think so, spirit?

ARIEL
Mine would, sir, were I human. (*The Tempest* 5.1)

This dialogue is the turning point of the play, Prospero's big "yoga moment." You can often hear a pin drop in the theater. The cycle of violence is stoppable by choice, right here and now. What will Prospero do? What would I do?

Prospero chooses the power of Patanjali's first yama, the yogic practice of ahimsa. He follows his spirit, his higher guidance:

Though with their high wrongs I am struck to th' quick,
Yet with my nobler reason 'gainst my fury
Do I take part. The rarer action is
In virtue than in vengeance. They being penitent,
The sole drift of my purpose doth extend
Not a frown further. (5.1)

Ahimsa is "the rarer action" at the heart of the play, the gateway to self-liberation in yoga, and incredibly beautiful to witness anywhere. If Prospero can do it, we can too. As Patanjali states and Shakespeare illustrates, compassion is what makes us truly strong and powerful. By forgiving others, we forgive ourselves. By loosening our false control over others, we free our souls.

Ahimsa doesn't mean we are doormats for evil and give in when necessary measures of defense are appropriate. Ahimsa is about engaging with the world without causing harm or injury, even during yoga class. When we know we are forcing a posture, the practice of ahimsa immediately recenters our mind-body connection. We can pause, breathe, and honorably feel the answer to the question: What is the most appropriate action right now? The necessary shift may momentarily trouble the ego, but it better ensures bodily safety and spiritual growth on the mat while fortifying our courage when we'll most need it for those "yoga moments" off the mat, including where ahimsa is most often needed—at home.

As American spiritual teacher Ram Dass is often quoted, "If you think you're enlightened, go visit your family." (Prospero does one better—he magically or mentally conveys his brother, political adversaries, *and* future-son-in-law *to him*, all in one go. What a multitasker!). Dealing with family, colleagues, rivals, self-identity, and the occasional visiting dignitary triggers the karmic emotional and mental patterning (samskaras) of many of Shakespeare's legendary characters. These same dynamics are often the underlying reasons we go to the mat: namely, to improve our relationships, usually beginning with our relationship with our body in some way: tighter abs, better range of motion, or lower blood pressure, for example. But whether it's with the people with whom we share our lives or what happens on the space of our yoga mat, it's all the same ahimsa practice, at home and abroad.

I don't think I'm the first yoga teacher to experience prolonged strife with a sibling. After twenty years of yoga, I still get my buttons pushed by a sister of mine. An argument of Shakespearean proportions can smack my inner world in an instant, signaling that a challenging "home practice" has begun. It's back to the mat and into my spiritual toolbox filled with Shakespearean yoga lessons. Thanks to yoga, I recognize that so much of the upset is simply a disturbing thought pattern (*vritti*) coloring *my* mind (*klishta*). It has absolutely nothing to do with my sister. Thanks to the Bard, I remember Prospero, Ariel, and the power of "the rarer action." My disquieted thoughts calm down the more I actively engage "my nobler reason 'gainst my fury." I regain my equilibrium more readily. Tempests subside with less upset, fewer tears, and a sincere effort to respond without creating more harm. Practicing virtue rather than vengeance feels harder to do than a series of yoga push-ups (*chaturanga*) at times; but Patanjali and Shakespeare give me every reason to practice, practice, practice.

Meanwhile, back on the island

Miranda, Prospero's sensitive daughter, is fully aware of her father's magical powers. She is Prospero's witness, and a very vocal one. As *The Tempest* opens, she believes her father's paranormal activity is clearly out of hand. Her first spoken line of the play is a plea for ahimsa: "If by your art, my dearest father, you have / Put the wild waters in this roar, allay them" (1.2).

"There's no harm done," he assures his daughter, twice. This repeated pledge suggests his machinations are of benevolent intent.

But it sure doesn't look that way.

The name Miranda is significant; it translates as "one worthy of admiration." She exudes natural compassion for those who suffer, in this case, at the hands of her father's rough magic, which currently seems to be running a very fine line between retaliation and resolution. Again, she cries:

O, I have suffered
With those that I saw suffer: a brave vessel,
Who had, no doubt, some noble creature in her,
Dash'd all to pieces. O, the cry did knock
Against my very heart. (1.2)

Ahimsa is often confused with love. We are all already essentially loving beings. Compassion is the practice of ahimsa that lets love flow. The word *compassion* breaks down as *com* (meaning "with") and *passion* (meaning "suffering" or "intense enthusiasm"). Miranda sees and feels deeply for people of her world (her dispute with Caliban's attempted rape being a valid one). Toward the end of the play, she proclaims:

> Oh, wonder!
> How many goodly creatures are there here!
> How beauteous mankind is! O brave new world,
> That has such people in 't! (5.2)

Miranda is more than Prospero's audience; her words acknowledge all of us, with our human capacity for beauty and bravery. We are those "goodly creatures." Highlighting this point, some actors playing Miranda visually embrace the audience with this passage, maximizing its poetic impact—and humor.

Miranda is also a superb exemplar for Patanjali's spiritual guidance on ahimsa in *Yoga Sutra* 1.33:

> To preserve openness of heart and calmness of mind, nurture
>   these attitudes:
> Kindness to those who are happy
> Compassion for those who are less fortunate
> Honor for those who embody noble qualities
> Equanimity to those whose actions oppose your values.[3]

Though tossed upon the seas, we change the world in wondrous ways when we rejoice for the smiling yoga student rising in Crow Pose (*bakasana*) while we teeter on bent arms; when we can be with our own suffering and use it as a way to connect to others who are also in pain; when we honor our brothers and sisters who serve humanity; and when, if discord strikes, we are still okay with another's right to an alternative opinion.

---

3. Nischala Joy Devi, trans., *The Secret Power of Yoga: A Woman's Guide to the Heart and Spirit of the Yoga Sutras* (New York: Three Rivers Press, 2007), 77.

Compassion and reverence for all beings moves us toward a universally happier ending. Voicing our truth on the violence we witness may not always be easy. But Shakespeare's plays illustrate that whether it takes five acts, five months, or five lifetimes, choosing virtue over vengeance is the ultimate divinity that shapes our ends.

A shelter from the storm

The title *The Tempest* is the perfect metaphor for the reason Patanjali imparts the sutras. Yoga calms the disturbances that cloud our peace (*yogas citta vritti nirodhah*, Yoga Sutra 1.2). A yogic interpretation of the play's title suggests that the real tempest is a raging fury inside the hero's mind. The day has come for Prospero to release his spirit and reclaim his rightful kingdom unfettered by the weight of guilt and retribution—emotionally and literally.

Shakespeare is an artful yoga teacher in the relationship between ahimsa and spiritual freedom. The quiet peace of our inner spirit (*purusha*) is the lighthouse whose beacon shines out over the thunder and lightning of our human drama, repeating, "Let it go. Let it go." Until we realize the storms we create of our own making, we are stuck, suffering and separated from our true Self. We are Prospero.

Ariel symbolizes Prospero's soulful inner guide (atman). This airy spirit repeatedly reminds Prospero that his freedom has been promised. He or she (nowadays, the role is often played as—and by—a woman) echoes Prospero's spiritual longing and Patanjali's reminder of what yoga will do for us: return our peace of mind. Ironically, Ariel possesses the inherent power to fly away anytime. She (or he) only *thinks* someone else can do it for her (or him), in this case a magician (the island guru) who is really just a symbol of the ever-present higher Self. So, too, our spirit longs for freedom, the promise of yoga. No one can do our practice for us.

As the final act unfolds, Prospero sets his spirit free. And the more Prospero surrenders his artful forms of control, the more he prospers. (His name—Spanish for *wealthy*—is no accident either.) Most important, it is he who now asks for forgiveness. He understands that "mercy itself . . . frees all faults," and sometimes it is our self we most need to forgive and release from mental bondage.

> Now my charms are all o'erthrown,
> And what strength I have's mine own
> [. . .]
> Mercy itself and frees all faults.
> As you from crimes would pardoned be,
> Let your indulgence set me free. (*The Tempest* Epilogue)

By the play's end, Prospero demonstrates that true power and strength come from within. He is also a much more likeable character. That friendliness Patanjali promises with the practice of ahimsa is apparent in him. The magician is humbly just a man again, yet a rightful ruler on his way home. So, too, *The Tempest* poetically mirrors our spiritual journey back to our peaceful center, that quiet place found in the eye of every storm. Our true home.

Accidental yogis

The transformative message of Prospero's words and actions is profoundly evident in the documentary film *Shakespeare Behind Bars*. As prisoner actors rehearse for a performance of *The Tempest*, interviews with the inmates reveal their personal learning curves. The lesson of forgiveness is foremost on their minds. One prisoner knows that he, like the character he plays (Prospero), has to work through the forgiveness process. He recognizes Ariel as his own mentor as much as Prospero's. Another inmate, initially cast as Antonio, honestly states, "The hardest damn thing I've had to do is forgive myself . . . . Sometimes the people who need it [forgiveness] may be the ones who deserve it the least."[4]

Likewise, Professor Laura Bates recalls her experiences of introducing Shakespeare to inmates of the Indiana prison system in her book *Shakespeare Saved My Life: Ten Years in Solitary Confinement With the Bard*. Like a good yoga teacher, she meets her students where they are—psychologically and quite literally, as detailed protocol protects her safe passage through corridors of barred inmates. She begins with passages and plays filled with criminality and punishment: the solitary confinement scene in *Richard II*, the magnetic lure of imagined daggers in *Macbeth*, and the theme of gang war in *Romeo and Juliet*. The first-hand insights these male convicts have into the psychological makeup of the characters rival those of any literary scholar or peace-loving yogi. For many of these prisoners, studying Shakespeare becomes a prized process, one that slowly reveals the mental and emotional afflictions (*kleshas*) that accompany violence, and the humility and enormous grace being human requires of us all.

The title of her book refers, in part, to inmate Larry Newton. He serves a life-sentence for the shooting of a nineteen-year-old college student walking his girlfriend home late at night in September 1994. By law, his sentence dictates no chance of a retrial or parole. It was that choice or the death penalty.

Through this inmate's intense dedication to comprehending Shakespeare, not only does he come to know his deed and his self more clearly, he inspires other prisoners to turn to the Bard for answers into who they are and for hope in who they can be. In correspondence with me, he writes what is true of Shakespeare (and, though unbeknownst to him, also true of yoga practice):

---

4. *Shakespeare Behind Bars*. Directed by Hank Rogerson (Kentucky: Philomath Films, 2005), DVD.

"Shakespeare has not changed my behavior. Shakespeare has simply inspired new thought, which in turn impacts behavior."[5]

Newton's act of taking a young man's life cannot be undone. Through Shakespeare, however, he has come to better understand how harmful thoughts and deeds are simultaneously universal and utterly avoidable. From his cell, Newton now writes Shakespeare courses for inmates. Like his teacher, he employs Shakespearean plays as an educational tool to raise awareness of the ultimate powerlessness of violence.

Depending on how you perceive Prospero's character, he, too, can be seen as a confined perpetrator of violence or an alienated victim of crime, or both. At both ends of the spectrum, ahimsa is necessary for healing and self-liberation. This is a spiritual process that is only as slow or as instantaneous as the ability of one's heart to dissolve the pain with inner light, like a fog in the sunshine (it took Prospero twelve years). But, as Shakespeare's yogis, knowing what we do about ahimsa, we are, hopefully, inspired to take those first steps toward reconciliation as soon as possible.

In prisons, schools, theaters, and anywhere Shakespeare gets people thinking about alternatives to violence, a positive ripple effect is set in motion. Patanjali tells us so:

> Being firmly grounded in non-violence creates an atmosphere in which others can let go of their hostility. (*Yoga Sutra* 2.35)[6]

It is no accident that Patanjali initiates us in the path of inner peace with ahimsa. This yama is an essential first step in preventing further suffering for ourselves and others. It is a way of thinking

---

5.   Larry Newton, letter to author, 6 July 2014.
6.   Hartranft, *Yoga-Sutra of Patanjali*, 35.

and being that embraces the inherent goodness in each of us. Because no matter who we are, what we've done, or where we find ourselves, going home to our true Self is the real magic.

CHAPTER 2
Shakespeare's Use of Violence to Highlight Ahimsa

There is no sure foundation set on blood;
No certain life achieved by others' death.
–King John 4.2

Any act that separates us from our Self, anyone, or anything feeds the ego—and is pretty messy. Shakespeare and Patanjali shed spiritual light on the effect of human violence and the deep, dark mental-emotional states that accompany it.

> We ourselves may act upon unwholesome thoughts, such as wanting to harm someone, or we may cause or condone them in others; unwholesome thoughts may arise from greed, anger, or delusion; they may be mild, moderate, or extreme; but they never cease to ripen into ignorance and suffering. This is why one must cultivate wholesome thoughts. (*Yoga Sutra* 2.34)[1]

By cultivating awareness, we come to recognize that any unloving, harmful, or violent act doesn't feel so good. We suffer and we cause others to suffer. Ahimsa unburdens our hearts and minds. It realigns the higher purpose of our yoga practice with our thoughts. We return to the surest foundation of life, the transformational strength and power of practicing ahimsa.

---

1. Hartranft, *Yoga-Sutra of Patanjali*, 33.

Messy stuff

Shakespeare is not your typical spiritual advisor when it comes to lessons on ahimsa. He purposefully puts our raucousness-loving egos on center stage with all the violence they generate. He hides nothing. Assassination, murder, suicide, execution, treason, war, and blood-spurting amputation of various body parts are all memorable scenes in the canon. *Titus Andronicus* contains the most notable loss of blood and a long list of characters seeping in basic moral ineptitude; Professor S. Clarke Hulse does the math: "14 killings, 9 of them onstage, 6 severed members, 1 rape (or 2 or 3, depending on how you count), 1 live burial, 1 case of insanity and 1 of cannibalism—an average of 5.2 atrocities per act, or one for every 97 lines." [2] Some critics suggest that *Titus* was the Bard's mockery of revenge plays. No matter what, audiences, both then and now, have packed the house fascinated by the soulless, useless cruelty the unchecked ego imparts in Shakespeare's tragic plays.

However, an important difference underscores Shakespeare's enactments of vehement mayhem and that of Hollywood's mega-million-dollar industry of gratuitous violence: intent. Rather than glorify violence or inspire more chaos and destruction, as many of today's blockbusters do, Shakespeare lowers the volume on the ego. How can that be?

Shakespearean audiences are privileged to both the inner thinking of his characters and the outward show of their actions. The mind-body connection is explored at an enormous level of depth that is rarely encountered elsewhere (with the notable exception of yoga philosophy). Privy to the rich and complex lives of Shakespeare's figures, we are vividly reminded what *not* to do when blame, guilt, jealously, and hatred flare up. Shakespeare

---

2. S. Clark Hulse, *Wresting the Alphabet: Oratory and Action in "Titus Andronicus"* (Detroit: Wayne State University Press, 1979), 106.

shows us his characters' tragic flaws, the errors and blind spots the characters themselves cannot see. The suffering we witness sobers us up. Our hearts awaken to the divine capability of nonharming, nonviolence, and mindfulness, given the same set of circumstances, because we recognize that violence could have been avoided. Aristotle labeled this empathic human reaction *catharsis*, a purifying or purging of our emotions after watching drama. Bruce Willis strikes me as a cool guy, but I just don't feel the same emotional cleanse after watching a *Die Hard* movie that I do after *Macbeth*, *Othello*, or *King Lear*. By contrast, Hollywood aims to keep us hooked, adrenaline pumped, and continually guessing: "Who done it?" The *why* is rarely examined. An often watered-down impact of bloodshed and massive destruction numbs our souls and exhausts our being.

By practicing ahimsa, we begin to choose more wisely how we spend our time and what constitutes wholesome visual input. The latent impressions that violence imprints on our consciousness must serve to further our spiritual journey rather than hinder it. In Shakespeare's day, the definition of "tragedy" meant the world would be rebuilt and order restored in some very painful way. Romeo and Juliet commit a double suicide, but the long-standing feud between the Montagues and the Capulets ceases (for the funeral rites, anyway); King Lear pays an unimaginably high price but learns moral lessons in human nature; in the same play, Gloucester is struck blind but gains inner sight; by the final scene in *Hamlet*, every major character is dead, but Hamlet has fulfilled his karmic duty and Fortinbras stands in the wings ready to restore political order. And let's not forget *Titus*. After all the horrific abominations, the one and only character to reform his bloodthirsty ways is elected Rome's leader. For any title character, Shakespearean tragedy guarantees death—physical, and perhaps more important, as a result of a harmful way of thinking or doing.

The price exacted for a character's particular vice bumping against *the* situation that fatally tests that character is our reawakening to the precious value of life. Shakespearean tragedy delivers more than sad endings; it is a purposeful lesson in the power of right living. No character survives violence unchecked. Hope is found in the cyclical mystery of nature, which always restores equilibrium. Our faith in a practice and in a theater experience of consciously examining our virtues and vices helps us and others to better avoid them.

Consciousness of ahimsa stems from a quiet, knowing peace within each of us, but more often than not, it's violence that gets our attention. The ego dramatically cries out, "Blame, guilt, abandonment, hate, and revenge!" This noisy seduction wants separation from what we perceive hurts or offends, cutting us off from our naturally peaceful selves and one another. Shakespeare's tragedies show that ahimsa is needed anytime the ego desires that separation rather than connection.

No laughing matter

When a character's radiant light of the Self is blinded and blackened by the ego, or when the hero's realization of a higher truth comes too late or not at all, we catch ourselves wiping away empathic tears. We relate to Shakespeare's most famous tragic characters because we know that we, too, unwittingly create whole scenarios brimming with judgment, revenge, self-aggrandizement, and escape. And it's all in our mind, even during our yoga practice. If we look serene on our mediation cushion but are simply rehashing our dislikes or justifying our retaliation of what someone "has done to us" (over and over and over), we feel anything but peaceful—just ask Hamlet, the self-tormented madman. (Macbeth knows something about what a mind "full of scorpions" feels like, too.) If we tell the truth only to destroy or disgrace another with our words, we, too, eventually become unhinged; in *Othello*, Iago's false truths are enough to earn him a first-class one-way ticket to hell (hell doesn't actually exist as a place in yoga, as no place really "exists" inherently, but you get the degree of evil that backfired on him). If we are consumed with critical thoughts about anything or anyone (our body, our boss, our bank accounts, etc.), our practice becomes merely a vain attempt to pacify our ego; King Lear takes a royal beating until he realizes the fragility of our existence and forgiveness.

Our human/god-like selves are still alive and well and playing themselves out onstage and on the mat. Both Shakespeare and yoga exist to lessen that struggle. The purpose of yoga is to return to our preexisting holistic being. Shakespeare shows how mental and emotional disturbances (vritti) hinder each hero, and us, quite differently. Doubt, guilt, misperception, imagination gone haywire, et cetera distract us from our higher purpose. It's our job as yogis to courageously wake up to our true selves and practice ahimsa when it's needed most. To clear our mind of the veils of illusion (kleshas). To choose the always timely option of nonharming. Ahimsa is the antidote, a way of life that chooses to connect to the good, best-intentioned, and spiritual aspects of others and, in turn, ourselves. When we replace unkindness, retribution, and hatred with wholesome thoughts and actions, our natural love shines through once again. We build our lives on the strongest foundation possible.

CHAPTER 3
The Timing of Ahimsa in Shakespeare's Plays

Our doubts are traitors
And make lose the good we oft might win
By fearing to attempt.
−Measure for Measure 1.4

The difference between tragedy and comedy is often the timing of ahimsa-related action.

Activating ahimsa

Shakespeare's comedies and late romances teach us that harmful acts only produce more hurt and separation, until the heart opens. Dr. Amanda Giguere's development of Colorado Shakespeare Festival's Shakespeare in the Schools Tour: Shakespeare and Violence Prevention has been nationally recognized. In 2011, she taught preventive messages about bullying in the local schools by staging Shakespeare's *Twelfth Night*, a funny and complex play that is also rich in yogic lessons on the cyclical nature of violence and the necessity of ahimsa. Post-play dialogue with students focused on Malvolio, a character teased and abused by those who love to hate his imperious demeanor. Having once played Maria, one of those bullies onstage, I reflected on my understanding of her actions from a yogic perspective after skyping with Giguere (more on that in just a bit).

The Malvolio subplot is a great example of the way a power imbalance can initiate the cyclical nature of violent behavior.

Malvolio is the head steward in Olivia's household, where, at present, a festive lot of zanies are camping out. For sport, by dropping a forged letter in his path, they lead him to believe he is beloved of his mistress. He takes the bait and experiences humiliations that make everyone—onstage and off—laugh, but with a growing discomfort as the play unfolds. The increasingly mean-spirited downfall thrust on him is an experience in ahimsa that also touches our hearts. Malvolio's transformation has the ability to transform *us* too. We shift to compassion for the universality of his experience and respect for his endurance of notorious abuse. But is it too late? Shakespeare suggests the cycle of violence never ends unless we act. Patanjali concurs. In *Yoga Sutra* 2.35, he states:

> When non-violence in speech, thought and action is established, one's aggressive nature is relinquished and others abandon hostility in one's presence.[1]

The Colorado Shakespeare Festival educator (who is also an avid yogini) highlighted the Malvolio subplot to illustrate how easily we become bystanders to bullying. She pointed out, "As audience to the unchecked exploits against Malvolio, we can consider ourselves likewise (unwittingly) responsible for the cyclical nature of more violence when he delivers his pointed parting line, 'I'll be revenged on the whole pack of you' (*Twelfth Night* 5.1). Especially when an actor playing Malvolio includes a direct gaze at the entire audience sounding his revenge, Shakespeare shows how easy it is to become complicit in harmful behavior."[2] During our call, Giguere held up a large white sign that read: "By being an 'upstander' bullying is stopped 57% of the time." Those can be less than desirable odds that put our yogic practice to work! (This is especially true if you work in Regan's household in *King Lear*.

---

1. Iyengar, *Light on the Yoga Sutras of Patanjali*, 149.
2. Dr. Amanda Giguere, interview with author, 13 October 2014.

Regan is one of Lear's two sinister daughters; when a guard pro-
tests her senseless order of the nobleman Gloucester's death, she
kills him on the spot.) It takes conscience and courage to activate
the potential for change anytime we witness the cycle of violence
being perpetuated. Ahimsa is a large part of that transformational
practice. Any time we can help prevent violence, if even in our
desire to have it cease, we are practicing yoga, Patanjali says:

> The desire to act upon unwholesome thoughts or actions
> or to cause or condone others towards these thoughts or
> actions is preventable. (*Yoga Sutra* 2.34)[3]

A problem like Maria

Yoga was not quite mainstream in the summer of 1987. At the
time, if asked, I would have blankly responded, "Patanjali who?
Yoga what?" Over twenty-eight years have passed since I played
Maria, and yoga is now a way of life for me and millions more. The
one thing that remains the same is the weird uneasiness I felt as
the play progressed; it also explains why Maria simply disappears
from stage, out of work and destined to marry Olivia's drunkard
uncle, Sir Toby Belch. Yoga has helped me better understand the
quality of character transference I felt as the joke went too far and
greater separation occurred.

Maria is everything Malvolio is not. She's clever and vivacious,
easily persuaded to cast aside her duties as Olivia's hired confidant
to party with visiting family, a growing number of friends of visiting family, and a fool named Feste. It is she who devises the plot
to revenge Malvolio's irksome and hypercritical mannerisms, and
the party loves her for it. Playing Maria was fun, no doubt about
it. I sashayed in an apple-red dress, stepping onstage with the sole
purpose of having a good time. It was a welcomed relief from the

---

3. Devi, *Secret Power of Yoga*, 175.

isolation and sorrow of playing Lady Capulet in *Romeo and Juliet* the previous summer, and I was sorry when the performances ended for the year.

Maria's role abruptly ends in Act 4, just as the darkest, meanest exploits are perpetrated on Malvolio. I generally spent most of Act 5 sprawled long on a wooden bench under the pecan trees located on the side of the open-air theater barn. Voices carried all too well. I listened to Malvolio bemoaning his plight and, soon thereafter, promising his revenge. I had had my fun but it left me somehow unsatisfied, cut off from the action and feeling a bit guilty. How else do I self-inflict separation from others through harmful words or behavior? How often do I unconsciously induce or watch suffering but feel disconnected from it? It was Maria, my character, not I, who did that to Malvolio. Or was I complicit as the performer? To play Maria again, I would take pause. I would consider the cycle of violence I was to set in motion, and my performance would no doubt alter with increased awareness of accountability. Shakespeare is all for a good laugh at our human vices, including Malvolio's (which is to be too full of self-love, or *asmita*, as it's called in yoga philosophy). But he also teaches a spiritual lesson: when the intent is to harm and spins out of control, a price will be paid. The cost of immoral behavior depends on the severity of the harm done and how quickly measures are taken to stop violence from being perpetuated. Ultimately, both yoga and Shakespeare help us see our role as yogis as first and foremost being to do no harm, to ourselves or others. When we are conscious of the yoga practice of ahimsa, our every thought, word, and action helps stop and reverse the cyclical nature of violence; without it, suffering strikes, again and again.

Standing up to injustice takes courage; voicing our concerns for those in pain takes bravery. But when being more conscious of living without causing harm to others is our daily—sometimes moment-to-moment—intention, we silence the doubts that would otherwise betray the good our yoga practice can really do in uniting our spirits.

Satya

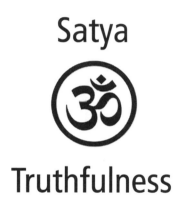

Truthfulness

CHAPTER 4
Satya as Reflected in *Hamlet*

Words, words, words.
—Hamlet 2.2

Our choice of words shapes our lives. The power of truthfulness and integrity to manifest our words into reality is the second yama of the Eight-Limb Path, a practice called satya. There are several other notable English interpretations derived from the Sanskrit term *satya*, including "unchangeable" and "reality." Shakespeare, a—if not *the*—literary master of the English language, emphasizes the vital impact words play in understanding how we perceive our reality. Being honest—the essence of satya—is a repeatedly prized virtue in Shakespearean characters. In key plays, silence—another aspect of satya—influences the course of events in profound and thought-provoking ways. Deception—the absence of satya—depends on the intention of the speaker. Commonly used plot devices involving deception are comical when intention is benign; but, in the hands of his villains, deception, including lying and slander, ranks as one of the most destructive and deadly vices. Applying Shakespeare's yogic lessons on how we communicate, including how we talk to ourselves, increases our awareness of Patanjali's one and only sutra on satya:

> Dedicated to truth and integrity (satya), our thoughts, words and actions gain the power to manifest. (*Yoga Sutra* 2.36)[1]

---

1. Devi, *Secret Power of Yoga*, 184.

Satya is a multifaceted practice, one that is felt as much as it is heard or seen. Patanjali promises that when we are dedicated to satya our thoughts, words, and actions become more easily realized. Our unspoken words are therefore just as important as those we consciously verbalize. Satya also includes trusting our intuition when information appears misleading. By witnessing the way thoughts become words and words become action, we are reminded that only communication that is in alignment with ahimsa (nonharming) puts the heart to rest.

Yoga strengthens our ability to be conscious communicators. We become aware that more listening and less talking often yields better results; that actions preach louder than words (just ask your kids); and that any communication must be thoughtful, true, and necessary if we are to positively reach our audience as speakers, teachers, writers, and community leaders. Everything else eventually collapses under the weight of lies and the energetic overload of inauthenticity.

Some of the Bard's most (in)famous characters and memorable plots are deeply moving explorations into the nature of satya. What determines comedy or tragedy is a hero(ine)'s ability to speak, hear, see, and intuit the truth before it's too late. Their trials and self-growth are our valuable lessons in the pivotal role that right speech plays in the practice of everyday enlightened living.

What's up?

Hamlet is a prince who questions everything—at length. In weighing his answers, often aloud to himself (for our benefit), he speaks 29,551 words over the course of what is the longest Shakespearean play.[2] Questions abound from the very first line of the play: "Who's there?" quickly followed by "What, has this

---

2. http://www.shakespeare-online.com/faq/shakespearelongestp.html. Based on the first edition of *The Riverside Shakespeare* (Boston: Houghton Miller, 1974).

thing appear'd again to-night? . . . Is it not like the King? . . . Shall I strike at it with my partisan [a weapon with a long shaft]?" As the audience, you immediately get the idea that the Elsinore guards seek answers to a very problematic situation (which happens to be about the ghost of Hamlet's father lurking about the castle at night and what action should be taken). By the time we get to Hamlet himself, we are well prepared for the most famous question of all time: "To be or not be?" And, like the guards, his verbal self-examination goes on to question what action to take:

> Whether 'tis nobler in the mind to suffer
> The slings and arrows of outrageous fortune,
> Or to take arms against a sea of troubles
> And by opposing end them. (*Hamlet* 3.1)

Hamlet intuited that something strange and unnatural was behind his father's death. Once the truth of his prophetic soul is confirmed, what he feels compelled to do about it thoroughly confounds him. The ineffectiveness of self-doubt rules his inner and outer kingdom. Hamlet says one thing but does another. He broods. He hesitates. He chooses to act out rather than to be direct and authentically himself. His life remains tormented. The internal chatter in his head simply overwhelms him. In this respect, Hamlet and Arjuna from the Bhagavad Gita would make fast friends. They both wrangle with existential issues as they strive to ignite right duty against the inner dynamics of self-doubt and familial loyalty.

His murderous, usurping uncle, Claudius, has similar difficulties. His prayers fly up but his thoughts of getting away with it all remain below. It's no wonder things are rotten in Denmark. For all their talk, commitment is lacking. Satya teaches us that, to be effective, thoughts, words, and actions must align with integrity. And they clearly do not in Elsinore. Honesty is sorely lacking and deception is stressing everyone out. I don't think a spoiler alert is necessary before telling you the entire clan ends up in a pretty bad way—and the truth prevails, albeit painfully and poignantly.

Tuning in

A great deal of satya is about refining the channel to which our internal dialogue is tuned. In yoga class, I often remind students to tune in to "radio you." By slowing down, regulating the breath, and observing thoughts without attachment to outcome, we make the truth of any matter more readily available. We start to discern fact from opinion, unfounded fears from ego-influenced garbage, inspiration from a complete waste of time. Intent to be open to the truth centers us. The inner teacher (atman) becomes undeniable and clear. There is a distinct feeling of "aha" behind the direction we receive in this receptive state, because the truth of the matter and the action one feels prompted to take are heartfelt. When internal chatter is indecisive and opens fire with more questions, the mentally based response only muddles the mind space more. In our gut, we sense something is off. Paralysis by analysis sets in. Like Hamlet, we may not always like the internal guidance we know and feel to be true, but the information flowing from our true Self remains unchangeable, the truth of our reality, nonetheless. Yoga is about setting the truth in motion. It is a philosophy of right action that aligns satya with ahimsa to elevate our lives and the lives of those around us.

Clear lines of communication

It takes about an hour, the average length of a yoga class, for the adult mind to quiet down. As a writer, I have known some of my best ideas to bubble up during yoga practice. Titles, sentence construction, and inspiration arise not because I'm trying to figure things out during Seated Forward Bend (*paschimottanasana*), but because I am *not*. Yoga naturally opens the mind as it lengthens limbs and brightens blood flow. Such inspirational moments may feel like a surprising gift, but they are perfectly natural by-products of satya, receptivity to the truth by quieting the mind. Struggle is replaced with the clarity of "Yes, that's it."

Helpful inspiration that rings true is relatively easy to actualize. Truths that clearly advise us it's time to change something about our life, our partnership, or our yoga practice, especially situations that strike us as uncomfortable or downright painful, are a bit stickier—as Hamlet demonstrates all too well. When yoga practice stirs up challenges that test our practice of satya, we want to watch and learn from the great Dane's resistance to the truth. Are we honest with our abilities on the mat? Do we follow through with the necessary discipline to do our practice regularly? Or do we just talk about it? When the voice of inner guidance speaks, do we listen?

Practicing what we preach

I have sweat buckets full of dedication to a hot yoga practice for over twenty years. My husband and I eventually opened a studio, and that one grew into three. A lot of happy, sweaty people found wellness and community under our care, and the businesses thrived. Eight years into the enterprise, a shift in my health arose. I felt unusually tired and my left arm starting shaking toward the end of classes. I sought the advice of doctors, neurologists, and, above all, my trusted practitioner of TCM (Traditional Chinese Medicine). It was she who, gently but firmly, confirmed—"O my prophetic soul!" (*Hamlet* 1.5)—that I should not subject my changing constitution to sweating (or stress) as much as I was. Like Hamlet, my mental chatter resisted satya in a thousand shades of fear and self-punishment (disturbing thought patterns Patanjali labels vritti): *But my practice? My livelihood? My community?* . . .

vritti, vritti, vritti. These thought patterns were upsetting me in a big way because I was clinging to and identifying with them.

As a studio owner, I have several times witnessed new students dive into a yoga regime, make remarkable strides, exclaim how amazing they feel, then suddenly quit. One such student called me confessing she couldn't handle the life changes she felt the practice was stirring up in her. She cried and I listened. Yoga has been around for thousands of years. It will be there still, if and when she decides to return to the mat. So, too, the truth of her necessary changes will continue to make themselves known in one or another way, shape, or form. It is my hope she has found a practice that guides those changes in a timely and gentle manner. She certainly came to mind when I was confronted by the truth my own practice stirred up. A major change was clearly needed and I felt the hefty power of satya at work.

I am happy to report that my asana practice is a lot slower and less sweaty these days; our talented teachers now own the still-thriving studios; and I am on to a new occupation better suited to my body's changing needs: writing, something I've longed to do for decades. My awareness of the importance of recognizing and activating the honest truth my soul imparts has heightened thanks to *Yoga Sutra* 2.36 and Shakespeare's *Hamlet*.

Famous last words

When it comes to satya, Hamlet's dying words (three hours later) are hard-won yogic wisdom. The prince fades, saying, "The rest is silence" (5.2). In his fleeting last moment, a peace floods his quieted soul. His many questions have been answered, his karmic duty is fulfilled, and, in the most painful way possible, he has exhausted any resistance to speaking or acknowledging the truth. Actors playing Hamlet often comment on the palpable spiritual release they experience delivering this final line.

Although Shakespeare officially extends the play with additional short speeches (and another line of questioning from Fortinbras), some directors purposefully end the play on Horatio's two lines just following: "Now cracks a noble heart.—Good night, sweet prince, / And flights of angels sing thee to thy rest!" (5.2).

When signaling Corpse Pose (final *savasana*) at the end of a yoga class, I am known to quote Hamlet's famous last words and Horatio's farewell. I encourage students to be content to rest in silence. To let their hearts break open and hear the angels sing. To let the music of satya be heard and felt in every blissful moment of nothing to say, nothing to do, nothing to question.

Simply be, allowing your soul to be at peace with truth of who you really are.

CHAPTER 5
Satya as Reflected in *King Lear*

Love, and be silent.
–King Lear 1.1

As we progress on the path of spiritual development, we become better communicators—usually that means talking less and listening more. Our hearts awaken to the vibrational power of sound, and we become more adept and more discerning in our use of words and language to convey what serves the highest good. In some cases, that means saying nothing. In other instances, we speak our truth, as withholding our knowledge would cause more harm to ourselves or others. Throughout Shakespeare's plays and during our yoga practice, the purposeful use of silence speaks volumes and, if not handled with care, can be radically misunderstood. Cordelia, the youngest daughter in *King Lear*, is a provocative example, showing that the practice of satya is not always easy or clear-cut, especially when it comes to speaking from the heart and allowing actions to speak louder than words. To some, she stands as the paragon of satya; others, however, question her motive and her skillfulness in delivering the searing truth. In the same play, fools teach wisdom and antagonists appreciate the fact that our speech has the power to do good in the world. Once again, Shakespeare lays wide open the spiritual lesson and leaves the many aspects of the truth to speak for themselves.

An inconvenient truth

Language and communication themes and motifs involving satya permeate *King Lear*. The play opens with gossiping noblemen, quickly followed by the all-too-common circumstances of a heated family discussion, one in which every word counts. As the aging king publicly prepares to divide his vast lands amongst his three daughters, he poses a weighty question: "Which of you shall we say doth love us most?" (*King Lear* 1.1).

Now, as one of three daughters myself, if I heard my gray-haired dad ask this same question at the next family reunion, my mouth would drop open. "Really?"

But that is exactly what Lear asks, the question itself boding the beginning of his downfall due to *hubris* (Aristotle's term for "pride" or "arrogance"). The daughters' answers quickly further the drama. Goneril, the eldest daughter (whom I've played onstage), lays it on. In courtly, measured speech she falsely flatters the king, her father, and, as a result, riches are heaped upon her.

As Cordelia ponders her turn at the podium, she asides, "What shall Cordelia do? / Love, and be silent" (1.1).

Cordelia's use of the word "do" rather than "say" highlights the fact that, so far in the conversation, words have cheapened love and only served to puff up Lear's ego. Cordelia consciously plans to communicate her take on the matter quite differently—with action and notably few words.

Lear's second daughter, Regan, plays her father's game all too well. She responds even more effusively than her older sister and Lear generously bestows upon her an ample third of his fair kingdom. Cordelia reassures herself once again:

> Then poor Cordelia!
> And yet not so; since, I am sure, my love's
> More richer than my tongue.

Cordelia's turn finally arises. "Speak," Lear commands.

CORDELIA
Nothing, my lord.

KING LEAR
Nothing!

CORDELIA
Nothing.

The situation grows increasingly awkward. Perhaps he thinks his favorite daughter is being shy or doesn't understand what's at stake? Her overdue response is no joking matter.

KING LEAR
Nothing will come of nothing: speak again.

CORDELIA
Unhappy that I am, I cannot heave
My heart into my mouth: I love your majesty
According to my bond; no more nor less. (1.1)

Cordelia's silence is not so much in words, but rather in the fact that she won't participate in the "glib and oily" adoration contest, one she finds impossible and unworthy of the love she truly feels for her father. Her response echoes Mark Anthony's opening volley to Cleopatra in the play Shakespeare wrote within a year following *King Lear* (1606–7 for those tracking the Bard's chronology):

CLEOPATRA
If it be love indeed, tell me how much.

MARK ANTONY
There's beggary in the love that can be reckon'd [counted]. (*Antony and Cleopatra* 1.1)

Antony and Cleopatra have their own serious issues with love and language, romantic though they may first strike us. For Lear's part, unfortunately, he proves to be morally blind and misjudges everything spoken—or purposefully unspoken—by all his daughters. The truth of his faithful daughter's reasoning falls on his deaf ears. Lear, infuriated, disappointed, and no doubt feeling publicly embarrassed, rashly disowns Cordelia. To make matters worse, he also kicks out his loyal servant Kent for agreeing with her. Disinherited, Cordelia departs with the King of France, who, astutely, appreciates the integrity Cordelia demonstrates during this tacky love Q & A. By the end of this emblematic opening scene, Lear's inner world begins to unravel. And, like anyone not willing to accept or hear the truth, he suffers the consequences greatly.

Audience to this family drama, we ask ourselves: Could both father and daughter have communicated more skillfully? Is Cordelia's refusal to answer the question well intended, but her limited response and timing missing the mark? Does Lear protect his pride at the expense of isolating those who refuse to pander to his ego's unquenchable need for special love?

Some directors follow the "apple doesn't fall far from the tree" theory: Cordelia is simply as stubborn and controlling as her father. She is a reflection of Lear. This interpretation is certainly a plausible take on the situation, although it doesn't fully explain Cordelia's motive. It also masks the courage of her authenticity, reducing her to simply a product of her environment, one that is choking in a web of lies. Shakespeare's enduring brilliance radiates from the open-ended interpretations of such provocative and timeless human experiences—in this case, issues surrounding satya, spiritual lessons in honesty and integrity that are as pertinent to a king and a princess as they are of our practice of conscious living.

The heart of the matter

Mahatma Gandhi said, "Truth resides in every human heart, and one has to search for it there, and to be guided by truth as one sees it. But no one has a right to coerce others to act according to his own view of truth."[1] The heart is the seat of pure knowledge, for which Cordelia is well named. Her name stems from the Latin *cor* or *cordis* (meaning "heart"). Moreover, in French, the word for "heart" is *coeur*, from which we get the term *courageous*. From a spiritual perspective, she exemplifies Gandhi's reflections on truth: she is courageously guided by the heart's wisdom.

Patanjali also tells us of the importance of heart-centered guidance: Focusing with perfect discipline on the heart, one understands the nature of consciousness. (*Yoga Sutra* 3.35)[2]

From the vantage point of the *Yoga Sutras* and the human energy systems they activate, love glows like a flame in the heart, the energetic nexus of soundless sound (*anahata* chakra). It is therefore not surprising that Cordelia says, "I can not heave my heart into my mouth" (*King Lear* 1.1). She naturally understands that love radiates from the heart as a vibration of indivisible union. Words fail to accurately express the human emotion of love (although Shakespeare himself certainly tries on occasion). It is no wonder that Cordelia cannot (or will not) articulate her love. To do so would only further her father's illusion that love can be made quantifiable. She would rather say nothing than disingenuously equate love in terms of material property. Nor does she want to further her father's self-deception; her enterprising sisters have already done a right fine job of that. Most important, she doesn't view his error as real and therefore doesn't try to defend herself

---

1. K. Kripalani, ed., *All Men Are Brothers: Life and Thoughts of Mahatma Gandhi as Told in His Own Words* (Paris: UNESCO, 1969), 71.
2. Hartranft, *Yoga-Sutra of Patanjali*, 53.

when stripped of an inheritance, nor does she try to make Lear feel guilty for his mindless, reactionary behavior. She trusts the truth and that the results will take care of themselves. This is how a yogin or yogini acts.

Cordelia does not appear again until late in Act 4, but she never stops loving Lear; severing their bond is, spiritually, not possible. When father and daughter are reunited (offstage), a witness to the scene reports that Cordelia was so overwhelmed with pity and love by her father's dire transformation that she cried smiling, her face a mixture of "sunshine and rain at once" (4.3). They are together onstage when Lear asks for her forgiveness. Cordelia responds with a spiritual awareness of the human illusion (maya) of separation and the burden of guilt that the human experience associates with it. She tells her father, "No cause, no cause," meaning she has never blamed him, nor will she. She knows there is nothing he—or anyone, including her deluded sisters—can do that will ultimately change our divine interconnectedness.

Truth or dare?

Cordelia's compassion and refusal to participate in her father's foolish love contest equate to a gentle patience that endures throughout the play. But is her excessive emphasis on the truth any less tragic than her father's folly?

Aristotle would say no. A hero or heroine's tragic downfall is often due to an imperfection in character, including positive forms of excess. In Cordelia's case, her adamant refusal to be anything less than honest initiates a painful process of self-awakening for both father and daughter.

Satya is an ethical inquiry that both Shakespeare and Patanjali leave open to interpretation. Patanjali's take on satya is clearly one of restraint (hence a yama). It is a daily practice of honesty and integrity needed for spiritual growth. Truthfulness requires awareness, which, in turn, unveils powerful insights into our consciousness. Shakespeare's presentation of Cordelia is of a mature woman who consciously examines her heart for the truth before she speaks. And, as is so often the case, her honesty and authenticity raise more questions than answers. Ultimately, there is no one but us ourselves to say whose take on Cordelia's truthfulness is the most correct. What is consistent throughout Shakespeare's plays and the sutras, though, is that the spoken and unspoken aspects of our every communication deserve mindful consideration.

Applying this lesson to the yoga experience, do we likewise pause to consider the ramifications of voicing our truth? Can we refrain from articulating an opinion, rebuttal, or defensive statement that may be factually accurate but ultimately harmful if spoken too soon, or at all? Can we recognize when speaking the truth means saying nothing? Are we willing to patiently wait for self-awareness to mature and evolve without putting anyone, including ourselves, on a guilt trip? Do we spin conversations that demand proof that we are special or the most correct? Are we comfortable in trusting the process? As with Mahatma Gandhi, standing by the truth for the greater good often requires accepting the painful personal consequences that may follow. Life is not always easy or convenient. There are gray areas that must be considered and weighed carefully. Doing or saying nothing until our heart is clear and unfettered by emotion or the fear of consequences is difficult, especially in a growingly impatient world where efficiency and effectiveness are not always balanced.

Be careful what you wish for

Shakespeare's *King Lear* confirms Patanjali's sutra insofar as the truth of our words bears fruit. Lear's words manifest exactly as he tells Cordelia in Act 1: "Nothing will come of nothing." As the play progresses, he is systematically dismantled from king to wandering madman to nothing, and he dies. Cordelia's words also manifest. "Nothing" describes her father's future as much as it does her own (and ours, as well), though hers is one she is perhaps more spiritually comfortable in accepting.

My study of the *Yoga Sutras* and the recurring importance Shakespeare puts on language has greatly influenced my more conscious choice of words over the years. I am much more aware of the importance of speaking positively and limiting any coarse language, especially when I'm tired or angry. I talk as if the Universal Power is listening. Understanding the power of our thoughts and words to manifest, I immediately notice when someone describes their life, body, or practice in negative terms. Whether or not I say something depends on my relationship with the person and the timing and circumstances of the situation. We all need to vent on occasion, but when someone's speech is a continual barrage of negativity, there is an underlying unhappiness. If my husband or I say something negative or unkind, one immediately corrects the other with the words "cancel, cancel." It is amazing how this short phrase diffuses any emotional negativity with a little levity and realigns our awareness with the power of satya.

Our yoga toolbox

Breathing exercises (pranayama) are an invaluable tool for calming our emotions and clearing our head when we are faced with circumstances that may courageously test our own practice of satya. International yoga teacher and author of *The Breathing Book* Donna Farhi says, "There is truthfulness to the breath." She explains, "When I listen to the intelligence of the breath, I feel I am being guided by something much more reliable than my mind, my ego, or my ambition."[3] Practicing yoga includes identifying when a patient and loving silence is our best answer. Yoga also teaches us that no amount of praise or money, and no number of awards, promotions, or pats on the back, will ever satisfy the precariousness of self-esteem built on ego. Only by recognizing the inherently divine nature of our perfect Self do we recognize our intrinsic worth.

Breath work is also an invaluable tool for centering our emotions and stabilizing our mental state. Quieting down enough to hear our breath simply roll in and out is brave and courageous work, especially in a society that seems increasingly uncomfortable with contemplation and "just being." Peace and quiet equates to boredom in much of today's world. A blank pause irritates egos fueled by advertising, the constant chatter of technology, and the race to respond to the ping of an incoming email or text. The skill needed to rise above the din of these distractions in order to hear the truth is needed more than ever. Breathing exercises improve our ability to hear the truth of our inner teacher (atman) while giving our desires, judgments, and opinions the opportunity to settle into their proper time and space. By listening to the truthfulness of the breath, we gain the moral guidance and the spiritual insight that come from making our way feelingly.

The teaching power of the Fool

Fools are often the wisest characters in Shakespeare's plays. They are the ones most likely to be in the present moment, commenting on any situation for what it is: a life lesson. When they speak, it will be the truth. The practice of satya is their role. Their ability to tell the truth with wit often makes us laugh, and it certainly makes us think twice. Take this example from one of

---

3.   Donna Farhi cited in Sam, "Yoga: To Breathe or Not to Breathe—There is no question," http://www.nimbingoodtimes.com/archive/pages2010/dec2010/NGT-1210-14-21.pdf.

Shakespeare's comedies: "The fool doth think he is wise, but the wise man knows himself to be a fool" (*As You Like It* 5.1).

Touchstone in *As You Like It*, Feste in *Twelfth Night*, and the Fool in *King Lear* are Shakespeare's great yoga teachers because they are not afraid of pushing buttons to skillfully inform and instruct. There is neutrality in the way they illuminate the cause of issues rather than further personal dramas. As great teachers, they know how to lighten things up when necessary by being foolish. Their authenticity captivates us because they hide nothing. They are willing to risk because they know there's nothing to hide. Likewise, a joyful honesty in our physical abilities during yoga practice, and appropriate, egoless feedback in our teacher-student dynamics is a sign our practice is working for us.

In *King Lear*, today's directors sometimes cast the same person to play Cordelia and the Fool. Shakespeare may have also double cast these roles; he conveniently, or purposefully, cues one to enter as the other departs. This doubling heightens the symbolic significance of having Cordelia and the Fool serve as ethical guides for the hero. Through their honesty or, as in the case of the Fool, darn-right frankness, they loyally stand by Lear's side, patiently witnessing his most painful moral education without judgment.

Double casting also highlights certain lines, such as "my poor fool is hanged" (*King Lear* 5.3). In yoga philosophy, the throat is the communication center (*vishuddhi* chakra). From this human energy perspective, it is highly emblematic that Cordelia dies by constriction at the throat. The term "fool" may imply that the Fool dies by hanging as well. I have seen a production of *King Lear* in which the director took Shakespeare at his word with that line, and the Fool was left hanging throughout intermission (pretty gruesome). Regardless of whether or not Shakespeare intended the line to pertain to just Cordelia or to also include the Fool, death by hanging spiritually symbolizes that living by the precepts of truthfulness, integrity, and authenticity are often extremely brave acts of courage.

The truth is out there

Thoughts and words matter and have the power to do great good. Shakespeare's many satya lessons in *King Lear* also include the power of speech to positively sway a villainous antagonist named Edmund from inflicting further harm. After being pretty much a jerk for the whole play, he is the one who attempts to save Cordelia and Lear from death in the eleventh hour, saying, "This speech of yours hath moved me, / And shall perchance do good" (5.3).

The truth is out there—in many forms. There are no pat answers. Stopping to think about the issues surrounding satya is the first step on the path to responsible speech. Our words reflect and have an impact on a collective thought system that we all share. It's our job to speak our truth in a wise and timely manner and abide by it from a place of love. Shakespeare's yoga highlights the way satya impacts our family relationships, our political arenas, and our personal practice of living a more conscious life for the good of all.

CHAPTER 6
Satya as Reflected in
Much Ado about Nothing

For man is but a giddy thing, and this is my conclusion.
—*Much Ado About Nothing* 5.4

Contrary to what today's audiences may generally think of as "gossip" or "gossiping," the terms had several different connotations in Shakespeare's day, the most frequent referring to "a close friend" or "a neighbor," as in *The Merry Wives of Windsor*, when one merry wife calls on the other saying, "What, ho, gossip Ford! What ho!" (6.2). Etymologists credit Shakespeare for coining the word "gossip" as a verb (with a positive connotation) to mean to "talk together" as close friends, as is twice heard in the closing lines of *The Comedy of Errors*: "With all my heart, I'll gossip at this feast . . . . Will you walk in to see their gossiping?" (5.1). Of Saxon derivation, the term "gossip" or "godsip" meant "God-parent." Some scholars say Shakespeare refers to the word's original associations with baptismal festivities in phrases such as "gossip's bowl" (*A Midsummer Night's Dream* 2.1, and *Romeo and Juliet* 3.5) and "gossip's feast" (meaning a christening) (*The Comedy of Errors* 5.1), as befits in Emilia's final line in *The Comedy of Errors*, "Go to a gossips' feast, and go with me. / After so long grief, such nativity!" (5.1). Every so often in his plays a "gossip" also denotes an idle chatterer, generally an old woman, but rarely one of malicious intent. Shakespeare's variable and evolving usage of the word "gossip" highlights his profound appreciation for the malleability of the human condition when language is involved.

Given the historical context of the word "gossip," a possible difference between gossip and slander is intent and integrity of speech, both aspects of satya (truthfulness). Gossip can be perfectly natural and harmless. Although the term is generally considered derogatory and associated with women these days, both genders use gossip as a way of passing along helpful advice, often of an intimate nature, to connect and create community. It is a process by which we are informed and entertained and it can reduce stress. Slander, on the other hand—or gossip turned malicious as it gets passed around, often misinterpreted—induces false rumor, doubt, and suspicion. It hurts and is hateful. The practice of satya is being mindful of what we say, and how and when we say it. As a result, satya better ensures that harmless gossip doesn't turn into harmful slander. It is a yama that also requires that we train our mind to see the truth of matters clearly lest we be led astray by those who make false and damaging statements about others.

Much Ado About Nothing is Shakespeare's "screwball comedy" all about the power of language to influence perception for better or worse. The difference between gossip and slander lies in the characters' practice of satya (integrity of speech)—or lack thereof. Shakespeare also examines the way that, even when there's absolutely nothing to what we hear or think we perceive, our imaginations can make fools of us and in some cases induce suffering.

Smoke and mirrors

If we were to listen in on a conversation from the late sixteenth century, the word "nothing" would sound like the word "noting" does to us today. And there's a whole lot of fuss over unsubstantiated reports of what is really going on in Messina, Italy, the setting for *Much Ado About Nothing*. It's a place where everyone is wrapped up in the latest news and eavesdropping but not always doing a very good job of getting their information straight. To intensify this contagion, in 2013, director Joss Whedon filmed his adaptation in a prestigious, modern-day mansion[1] architecturally packed with stairwells, nooks and crannies, and television security monitors primed for the false assumptions that arise by snooping around and noting only half of the story.

As the play opens, Leonato's household receives news from the warfront. A messenger reports that the prince, Don Pedro, and nearly all of his men are returning from battle unharmed and planning an extended visit. (It's a kind of *The Big Chill* scenario without the opening funeral procession.) As the reunion celebration unwinds, talk of war quickly turns to repartee on marriage versus bachelorhood. Claudio, the young war hero, has fallen head over heels in love with Leonato's only daughter and heir, Hero, and he asks his good friend Benedick and Don Pedro for their help in wooing her. Trouble is already brewing, however. Privy to these conversations, the prince's socially outcast brother, Don John, immediately plans to thwart Claudio's fun and games. He jealously feels that "that young start-up [Claudio] hath all the / glory of my overthrow" (*Much Ado About Nothing* 1.3), for no other reason than that's just the kind of guy he is. Don John is a self-proclaimed "plain-dealing villain" and a man "not of many words." When he does speak, it is for no good. For example, he puts a bug in Claudio's ear implying that the prince actually courts Hero for himself. Claudio is set straight on the matter, but he fails to learn the lessons in satya: not believing false rumor, especially from an unreliable source, and the importance of speaking for himself.

Don John quickly takes advantage of Claudio's gullibility again, this time while deceiving his brother, the prince, too by

---

1. The beautiful mansion happened to be the director's own house and the movie filmed in 12 days. As Hamlet would say in indie film circles, "Thrift, thrift, Horatio!"

adding something resembling visual proof (similar to the "ocular proof" that undoes the Moor in *Othello*). Borachio, Don John's coconspirator, arranges to be seen in Hero's bedroom window with a woman (Margaret) dressed up to look like Hero. Falling for this trick, Claudio publicly denounces Hero at the altar as a "rotten orange"—gasp!—and claims that her maiden modesty is a sham. This public slander is so ruinous to her honor that Hero faints. Friar Francis, a kind of well-intentioned spin doctor, wisely instructs the family to "pause awhile" and to report that Hero has died. Once Claudio (along with the prince) realizes the grievous fault, he will "resurrect" Hero.

The friar's instinct for patience proves spot-on. Thanks to some bumbling but ultimately effective watchmen, Don John's mean-spirited plot is soon brought to light. Ursula, Hero's gentlewoman, spreads the news:

> It is proved my Lady Hero hath been
> falsely accused, the prince and Claudio mightily
> abused; and Don John is the author of all. (5.2)

The truth prevails.

As part of Claudio's penance for "killing" Leonato's daughter, he will be fooled once again when he agrees to marry a woman of Leonato's choice. Perhaps Claudio's valiant war efforts boosted his karmic ratings, as his story ends well: he and the "new" Hero will indeed be happily wed while the slanderous instigator, Don John, is apprehended.

Despite the happy ending, Claudio serves as an example of the fact that believing everything you hear or think you see without reflection causes problems. His obsessive nature is the result of what Patanjali labels incorrect knowledge (*viparyaya*), or clouded thinking. Our senses are not the most reliable instruments of truth. Ironically, Claudio says as much during his verbal bloodbath of Hero in front of the wedding congregation: "O, what authority and show truth / Can cunning sin cover itself withal!" (6.1). Likewise, our imagination (*vikalpa*) often distorts reality; we can believe a bush is a bear, given the right circumstances. Memory (*smriti*) is often pitted with one-sided, emotionally charged impressions; and in deep sleep (*nidra*), our dreams lack the veracity of direct contact (unless of course you're Nick Bottom in *A Midsummer Night's Dream*, but even he concludes that his fantastical dream "hath no bottom" (4.1)). What could Claudio have done differently? How can we avoid his pitfalls when it comes to knowing and speaking the truth?

Testing, 1–2–3

Patanjali offers three ways to cultivate right knowledge (*pramana*), or unclouded thinking:

- make sure information is based on direct personal experience,
- put that information through a reasoning process, and
- validate it from a reliable source.

Also important is the understanding that all three aspects must be in agreement for you to recognize the truth. When they are, there's an undeniable sense that you know that you know. Or at least that you are on the right track to knowing.

> Knowledge embraces personal experience, inference, and insights from the wise. (*Yoga Sutra 1.7*)[2]

On top of a hefty dose of self-doubt and being quick to anger, Claudio lacked all three aspects of correct knowing: he did not actually see his fiancé that night; he jumped to conclusions; and

---

2. Devi, *Secret Power of Yoga*, 27.

he believed Don John, who, just a heartbeat ago, had proved he was not the most trustworthy source of information. Had Claudio stopped to examine his inferred thoughts before acting and speaking, he would have had a far more enjoyable premarital period. And what is prudent advice for a Shakespearean character is certainly good for us too!

Cupid's messengers

Whereas the Claudio-Hero plot is a heavy example of wrongly "noting" the situation, the play also contains a charming use of white lies. (This is one of Shakespeare's most popular comedies, after all.) Conspicuous gossip and revealing love notes become an entertaining game that draw Beatrice and Benedick together in love. Whether or not this is completely ethical is of course up for debate. But in yoga philosophy intention is everything, and the intention here is good. Several lines in the play indicate that Beatrice and Benedick have had a prior relationship. Beatrice alludes to as much while commenting on Benedick's affection, saying, "Indeed, my lord, he lent it me awhile; and I gave him use for it" (*Much Ado About Nothing* 2.1). Some productions, such as the previously mentioned Whedon contemporary adaptation, stage visual flashbacks of this implied relationship. Through these flashbacks and in the text itself we get a sense that their shared past was fervent but somehow not emotionally satisfying.

Beatrice is therefore always referring to Benedick as a "stuffed" and "pompous" man, insinuating he's a bit of a playboy; and Benedick is quick to verbally wrestle with her in clever defense for her ongoing commentary about his character. These are two sparring wits who are hiding their hearts behind wordplay and bruised egos. In short, they are the perfect match! Don Pedro and Leonato's family think so, anyway. They revel in conspiring to see them wed and eat their words expounding a bias for the single life. We are as overjoyed as the pranksters are in watching these two mature, intelligent, and ultimately loving partners overhear gossip intended to rekindle their passion and create a lasting bond. Well-intended "untruths" work to positively transform them, and, critical to the concept of satya, both Beatrice and Benedick come to know how it happened and still decide to stop talking long enough to kiss and marry.

Noisy news

Shakespeare's title couldn't be more apt. It's taken a whole lot of explanation to describe a plot about circumstances that were simply made up by the characters' ability to make other characters believe them. In German, *Much Ado About Nothing* translates as *Viel Lärm um Nichts*. The word *lärm* broadens the English translation of *ado* to include noise, din, racket, fuss, or alarm, all of which describe the effects of a play about faulty "noting." The play's title alone is valuable to our practice of conscious living: how often are we willing to admit that our personal melodramas and misperceptions are "full of sound and fury / Signifying nothing" (*Macbeth* 5.5)? When we stop and think about this question, we experience Shakespeare's yoga at play. Are we able to laugh at ourselves like Beatrice and Benedick when our words betray the truth of our hearts and crusty opinions? Can we ask forgiveness when our verbalized misperceptions cause duress, as Claudio did?

The practice of satya helps us to differentiate between harmful slander and harmless gossip in *Much Ado* and in leading an enlightened life. In his film commentary, Whedon shares what led him to making *Much Ado* in the first place: "Because of the darkness, because of the lying, because of the manipulation, because of the pain."[3] *Much Ado* addresses the need to include a wider range of possible truths at any given moment. For similar purposes, the

---

3. Commentary to *Much Ado About Nothing*, Directed by Joss Whedon (Los Angeles: Bellweather Pictures, 2013), DVD.

Colorado Shakespeare Festival in the Schools program has included this play as part of its educational outreach in promoting nonviolent behavior in schools. Director Amanda Giguere reports that *Much Ado* teaches kids about the negative effects of cyberslander—texting misleading images and withholding the truth. In the 2014 *Much Ado* adaptation she developed for the CSF in the Schools program, Claudio views a cell-phone "selfie" that has an imposter dressed up as Hero and locked in another's embrace. Giguere says, "*Much Ado* shows kids how every word, image and action impacts the entire school climate, and how Shakespeare is anchored in their world."[4]

Watching any version of *Much Ado* from a spiritual perspective accentuates the importance of truthfulness and integrity, as well as the disastrous results of lying, slander, and ill-intended deception; it also celebrates the joy of language and its power to heal and unite. The importance of sifting through critical details and checking our facts before nothing becomes something is vital to our health and that of our communities. It's one thing to enjoy *Much Ado*, as it's a very funny play; it's another to take the more serious messages peppered throughout and apply them to our lives in order to reduce prejudice, black-and-white thinking, and human misery caused by distorted truths.

Can we talk?

Applying satya to our yoga practice and studio policies requires the same kind of discrimination. As co-owner of a yoga studio in Wellington, New Zealand (the capital and entertainment hub of a small, beautiful nation), I assure you that the front desk supplied some of the best water-cooler talk in town. Politicians, noted healers, gurus, international yoga teachers, movie stars, dancers, singers, and everyday yogis from around the world

---

4. Dr. Amanda Giguere, interview with author, 13 October 2014.

leaned on the counter for information and conversation. I never knew whom I might meet on any given day. After classes, the desk was often swamped with happy, sweaty people asking questions and getting the latest scoop. Everyone was treated the same regardless of their celebrity status or longevity with the studio. We strived to make it a safe place where confidences were held and where people felt at home no matter who they were or what they were dealing with in life. This front-desk gossip was vital to our success. Local businesses such as ours grew by word-of-mouth more than by any slick ad. This giant "water cooler" also propagated an ideal environment for us to pass along the best healing practices, console sorrows, celebrate victories, laugh, and generally connect to a vibrant community of like-minded individuals. It was a place not unlike Messina. And we were not immune to our share of slander.

On one notable occasion, we encountered trouble. Our Don John appeared in the form of a visiting teacher. Although she glanced over the ethical agreement before teaching, she did not live by its principles, most especially those regarding confidentiality. Long story short, Claudio and Hero fared better than we did; no amount of explanation on my part could heal the breach her words caused. And I was saddened that I never saw the student affected again. An important lesson in satya was learned: the necessity of emphasizing the utmost need for confidentiality amongst the staff and in our student-teacher relationships. Moving forward, I made it a point to review aloud the ethical agreement line by line with any teacher or trainee that would be privy to information concerning any student, a confidentiality that inherently extended in or outside the studio environment. Integrity of speech includes refraining from causing harm to others by putting proper guidelines in place to ensure safe and clear lines of communication where we work and play.

Surface information versus in-depth reporting

Tabloid magazines, Facebook, and news media links circulate generalities about the lives of celebrities, politicians, and even our own affairs. These sources lead us to believe we know who these people really are and how our lives compare in some way, shape, or form. But do we? Wanting to know what's inside the minds of others, how they live, and what they wear, eat, think, or do is a compelling, timeless human pastime. We think that knowing all this will somehow make us feel better or at least entertain us for a fleeting moment.

Underneath this surface information, however, lies deeper wisdom: an understanding of the interplay between what Patanjali calls the seen and the seer. Several times throughout the *Yoga Sutras*, the sage advises us to separate any object, the seen (*prakriti*, which is changeable in nature, like our body and mind), from the seer (*purusha*, the soul or the true Self, which is pure awareness). The ability to tap into our wider lens loosens our attachments to the phenomenal world of appearances. As Friar Francis advises in *Much Ado*, satya teaches us to pause and consider where we may be blinded by false knowledge (*avidya*). We learn to recognize that what we note maybe nothing but projection (*adhyasa*). The practice of satya makes us feel more peaceful because we recognize that an unchangeable, divine awareness witnesses all perception. Of course, we have to make the best decisions we can with the information we have, or we would never get dressed in the morning. But when it comes to voicing and acting on our opinions and judgments, especially of others, it behooves us to listen and to learn from Shakespeare's dramatizations of our giddy nature and heed Patanjali's advice on the ways satya steadies our lives.

As a result, celebrity escapades, political scandals, and trivial personal affairs become less interesting while the relationship with our own inner guide (the seer) becomes more vital and more reliable. Satya reminds us that the impact of unpacking our hearts publicly comes with responsibility. The practice also enables us to be entertained and socially informed while maintaining a richer, wider worldview beyond headlines and first glances. Through this greater awareness, we learn that thinking for ourselves means slowing down to separate emotion from fact, fact from possibility of glossy fiction, and much ado from absolutely nothing to worry about.

Asteya

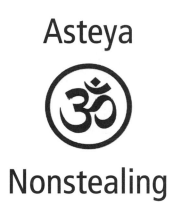

Nonstealing

CHAPTER 7
Shakespeare's Take on Asteya

Who steals my purse steals trash. 'Tis something, nothing:
'Twas mine, 'tis his, and has been slave to thousands.
But he that fliches from me my good name
Robs me of that which not enriches him
And makes me poor indeed.
—Othello 3.3

Positioned in the heart of the five yamas is asteya, restraint from stealing. You know you're on the right spiritual track in this regard when you are honest and generous with your time, resources, and energy. You believe and act as if there's enough for everyone. Practicing asteya also involves a dedication to dismantling the negative thoughts and destructive emotions that cause greed, jealousy, and prejudice. For, as you sow, so you shall reap. Patanjali explains:

> Abiding in generosity and honesty, material and spiritual prosperity is bestowed. (*Yoga Sutra* 2.37)[1]

Loss prevention

In Shakespeare's day "to steal" had a well-known variety of meanings. Characters could steal by taking or hiding something stealthily or by secretly withdrawing, as in creeping from one place to another. In either case there was often an accompanied sense of loss, seclusion, or deception that purposefully tried to stay hidden—but rarely did.

---

1. Devi, *Secret Power of Yoga*, 189.

Khaled Hosseini's book *The Kite Runner* emphatically stresses the importance of not stealing:

> (But) theft was the one unforgivable sin, the common denominator of all sins. *When you kill a man, you steal a life. You steal his wife's right to a husband, rob his children of a father. When you tell a lie, you steal someone's right to the truth. When you cheat, you steal the right to fairness.*[2]

Hosseini's clear and moving passage emphasizes the many types of theft that cause violence and suffering.[3] Shakespeare illustrates these many types of thievery, the mental machinations behind them, and their repercussions throughout the canon. Whether it's Claudius stealing the crown by killing his brother (*Hamlet*); Bardolph looting a French church after a war (*Henry V*); or Bardolph's drunkard role model, Falstaff, attempting to seduce someone else's wife (*The Merry Wives of Windsor*), a high price is paid for taking what is not rightfully one's own. These are Shakespeare's straightforward examples of the ethical importance of asteya.

The lessons of asteya played out on Shakespearean stage apply just as readily to basic yoga practice. If we are late to class, we steal the group's concentration and our own centered start to practice; if we lose our balance in Tree Pose (*vrksasana*) and berate ourselves, we undermine the yoga process by thinking transformation is a destination; asking to copy a teacher's music without giving the artist financial credit is piracy, plain and simple. Blame and justification doesn't get us anywhere. They only induce a vicious cycle of guilt and more blame, including self-condemnation and

---

2. Khaled Hosseini, *The Kite Runner* (New York: Riverhead Books, 2003), 106.
3. Yoga philosophy does not refer to stealing or any act of violence as "sin" per se. Rather, yoga aims to make us aware of the destructive emotions and distortions of thinking that induce such negative actions; they are called kleshas in Sanskrit and not considered part of our true nature.

spiritual unrest. Asteya is about becoming aware of any tendency to steal, including stealing from ourselves, however minor it may seem, and then making a sincere effort to refrain from such action.

So when the big rugs are pulled from underneath our feet— when we lose the job, the marriage dissolves, or unexpected news throws our fortunes into a tailspin, for example—we have internally prepared ourselves to turn inward, self-reflect, and carefully analyze what happened rather than steal the opportunity for self-growth. We practice asteya by refraining from throwing mud or laying on a personal guilt trip. And through asteya—lo and behold!—we immediately start to regain our equilibrium. Shakespeare echoes this fundamental yoga truth in *Othello* when the Duke of Venice counsels Desdemona's father, Brabantio, who is livid because his daughter has secretly married the Moor, Othello: "The robbed that smiles steals something from the thief, / He robs himself that spends a bootless grief" (*Othello* 1.3).

Shakespeare's yogic verses help us remember that no person nor any experience can steal our most valuable asset, our inherently peaceful center, unless we let them.

CHAPTER 8
Asteya as Reflected in *Othello*

No legacy is so rich as honesty.
–All's Well That Ends Well 3.3

"Honesty" is a word rich with multiple meanings in Shakespearean plays, including "not stealing," "sincere," and "chaste." In *Othello*, the Bard illustrates the importance of these definitions of honesty and how the appearance of honesty easily manipulates human behavior. When the play begins, Othello, a Moorish war hero, has it all: a loving wife, the glories of victorious battles, and radiant health. He resides in Venice after eloping with Desdemona, "a maid / That paragons description" (*Othello* 2.1), who represents what is good and noble in human nature. The tragedy is this: Othello proceeds to sabotage his marriage, career, and well-being by allowing his imagination to be malignantly twisted by Iago, who, although referred to as honest no less than fifteen times throughout the play, is clearly anything but that. Iago stands for everything that Desdemona does not, and Othello becomes lodged in soulful battle between the two forces: honesty and self-deception.

Iago serves Othello as his standard bearer and loathes him. "I hate the Moor!" Iago flatly admits, twice. And it is this hatred more than anything else that fuels his plan to destroy Othello from the inside out. Iago is a villainous artist, ingenious for his cunning ability to plant a series of loaded innuendos about his newlywed's faithfulness in Othello's brain. In Act 2, Iago unabashedly targets Othello with this devious plan:

[To] make the Moor thank me, love me, and reward me
For making him egregiously an ass
And practicing upon his peace and quiet
Even to madness. (2.1)

In a Portland Center Stage production of *Othello* (Oregon, 2014), audience members actually hissed at Iago as he laid out his psychopathic plot in soliloquy. (I joined in, just as any groundling paying one penny to see this same character in Shakespeare's own theater might have done.) Iago represents everything we fear to be true: that someone or something is out to steal our stuff, our position, our souls. If someone as brave and esteemed as Othello falls for Iago's seductive ploys, what's to save us from the same fate? The answer: yoga, ego-management (*atma vichara*), the one area of development Othello lacks.

Circumstances in Shakespeare's dramas that steal a character's peace of mind strike a deep note within us. They also reflect what is probably the most famous sutra, 1.2, which defines the very purpose of yoga: to find calm amidst the natural disturbances of the mind.[1] Other interpretations include to be able to find your equilibrium when external circumstances test your internal wisdom, and to be able to see clearly and truthfully in any situation and act accordingly. This is not easy work, and it may take lifetimes. It is also why theater patrons for centuries have identified so deeply with Othello's tragic flaw: a preoccupation with the appearance of things, which strips him of his "peace and quiet" and everything therein that is good and loving. His troublesome ego obscures the truth of who he and others truly are. He loses emotional, physical, and spiritual balance and his world unravels,

---

1. Edwin F. Bryant, trans., *The Yoga Sutras of Patanjali: A New Edition, Translation, and Commentary* (New York: North Point Press, 2009), 10-21.

quickly and disastrously. His is a self-inflicted theft crime that is entirely avoidable.

Although highly skilled at battling external enemies in the public realm, Othello (similar to Claudio in *Much Ado*), is completely unprepared for the private, internal war that rages in his consciousness as a result of evil misdirection of the truth. The name Othello contains the word "hell" and is an apt description of the depth of suffering that leads him to suffocate Desdemona and then take his own life. Othello's internal mental battle is our lesson in the pitfalls of self-sabotage, or stealing from our own well-being. Contrary to most traditional interpretations, Iago is not solely to blame. Othello primed himself for this particular karmic lesson in mental distraction and, unfortunately, learned the cause of his demise too late.

What's ego got to do with it?

Everything.

Through Othello's tragic downfall we reflect on the importance of mindfully managing the ego and not enabling anything or anyone to take our "peace and quiet" away, a primary yogic teaching. Because the word "ego" as we know it from modern psychology did not exist in Elizabethan speech (except when quoted from Latin, as in the phrase *Ego et Rex meus*, meaning "my king and I," which the Bard references in *Henry VIII* 3.2), one cannot help but marvel at Shakespeare's choice of the name Iago for his most crafty bad guy. Iago sounds remarkably like "I am ego." Whether or not this is yet another sign of Shakespeare's enlightened authorship, creative conjecture on my part, or simply coincidence, Iago symbolizes the ego, called *ahamkara* in Sanskrit, and its parasitical nature.

We need our ego for survival; it triggers fear, disgust, anger, and sadness, all of which have played a vital role in keeping us alive and evolving since the Pleistocene era. These same ego-driven emotions, however, also tend to negatively narrow our thinking and alter our already easily distorted perception. Our spiritual evolution depends on cultivating our higher consciousness and putting the ego in its rightful place and in constant check. Yoga guru B.K.S. Iyengar describes the ego this way: "It impersonates the self and acts as an impostor of the self. But it can also be transformed through practice to reach the sublime."[2]

Mindfulness training is key to coordinating the various functions of the mind to raise our awareness and avoid the living hell in which Othello finds himself as he woefully declares, "Farewell the tranquil mind" (*Othello* 3.3).

Iago personifies the voice of Othello's ego. Iago knows that his role is both parasitical and a selfish act: "I follow him [Othello] to serve my turn upon him" (1.1). This seemingly well-intentioned character knows what every person needs and the vices that drive those basic instincts to negative extremes. Iago's words fire unique emotional triggers and his schemes succeed because he "never knew a man who could love himself" (1.3). And Othello is no exception. He inwardly struggles with making the transition from his accomplished war-commander lifestyle to married life and Venetian customs. His self-image is under siege. He craves loyalty. In addition, those outward shows of success for which he has become accustomed and for which he has often been publicly praised are falling away. When Iago insinuates that Othello's bride is sleeping with his lieutenant, Cassio, a toxic mix of emotions set in: regret, anger, shame, and jealousy, all of which the ego magnetizes more easily under the duress of any major

---

2. Iyengar, *Core of the Yoga Sutras*, 190.

life transition. Othello becomes "perplexed in the extreme," and yet on some level he knows these disturbing thoughts are being driven by his ego (Iago). Throughout the play, the Moor rightly confronts Iago:

OTHELLO
By heaven, I'll know thy thoughts.

IAGO
You cannot, if my heart were in your hand;
Nor shall not, whilst 'tis in my custody. (3.3)

Iago's candid answers only drive Othello into deeper self-loathing because, of course, Iago is right: we are not able to read other people's minds. Reading one's own mind correctly is hard enough! This limiting insight is essential to the success of Iago's plot and likewise true of the hidden nature of the ego. The ego is out to serve the ego. It panders to our deceptive powers of perception (wrong knowing, imagination, dreams, sleep, etc.) unless we train the mind (*manas*) in correct knowing (*vidya*). Our ego's survival depends on always, always believing that our fear is real, that our sadness is perpetual, that our greed is justified, and so on. More often than not, however, these disturbing thoughts are just the unchecked ego pulling the ripcord on suffering. Unless unconditioned awareness steps in, clinging to the delusion of the solidarity of "my story" obscures the sight of one's divine nature, which can never be extinguished, since it is not subject to birth and death.

With each progressive wrong interpretation of what Iago (the ego) wants Othello to hear and see, Othello loses command of his higher consciousness. Symptoms of off-lining mental health set in: headaches, mumbled speech, and an onstage seizure. Patanjali's *Yoga Sutras* could have predicted as much:

Accompaniments to the mental distractions include distress, despair, trembling of the body, and disturbed breathing. (*Yoga Sutra* 1.31)[3]

Jealousy, the "green-eyed monster," methodically proceeds to eat Othello up, body and soul. Eventually, Othello states that his "heart has turned to stone" and commits himself to "put out the light"; his ego drives him to kill his bride and her reported lover. But, as Iago asserts at the tragic end, "I told him no more than he found to be apt and true" (*Othello* 5.2). In other words, Othello projected his own disturbing thoughts to justify his ego-driven actions. Iago did nothing but impersonate Othello's darkest self-doubts.

Our natural state is to be in awareness. When, like Othello, we are not in a state of awareness, then, Patanjali states, "the Seer appears to take on the form of the modifications of the mind field, taking on the identity of those thought patterns" (*Yoga Sutra* 1.4).[4]

It is Othello, not Iago, who took the bait, who saw what he wanted to see. He is not alone, either. Iago preys on most every main character's ego-centered soft spot: he pumps up Roderigo's lust for the now-spoken-for Desdemona, and subsequently Roderigo squanders his money and lands and eventually his life; Iago entices Othello's lieutenant, Cassio, to drink beyond his limit and get into a brawl, the consequences of which temporarily cost him his reputation; and Iago also persuades his wife, Emilia, to steal a prized handkerchief from Desdemona, and Emilia withholds this information when Othello emotionally abuses his bride for losing the love token. Iago stabs her. And even Desdemona, though loyal and true to her husband, accepts Iago's empathy and

3. Sri Swami Satchidananda, trans., *The Yoga Sutras of Patanjali* (Virginia, Integral Yoga Publications, 2012), 48.
4. Swami Jnaneshvara Bharati, "Yoga Sutras of Patanjali 1.1-1.4: What is Yoga?" SwamiJ.com, Accessed March 26, 2016, http://www.swamij.com/yo-ga-sutras-10104.htm

advice to be content, assuaging any guilt or regret she may harbor for deceiving her father while eloping. She dies too, though without recrimination, I might add. What Iago (the ego) tells Othello is true of every character, including us: "I am your own forever" (*Othello* 3.3). How we deal with the ego is Shakespeare's yoga lesson in asteya: the vital importance of not stealing from the truth of any situation. The use of deception to temporarily bolster our own self-worth backfires.

Know thyself

Othello locked his negative, ego-driven thoughts inside without a reality check on Iago's words. As a result he experiences a spiritual identity crisis. If Othello had given Desdemona the opportunity to dispute the allegations straight away, confronted Cassio, or simply trusted his higher reasoning, tragedy could have been avoided and Iago exposed. But, as in our own push-pull relationship with the ego, these were personal matters he was unwilling to explore or uncomfortable doing so. In Oliver Parker's film adaptation of *Othello* (1995), the title character (played by Laurence Fishburne) literally submerges Iago (played by Kenneth Branaugh) under ocean waves, threatening to kill him if his insinuations about Desdemona prove false. The visual metaphor brilliantly illustrates Othello's efforts to push his ego-propelled, disturbing thoughts deep down inside his self, though they keep resurfacing intact.

Acquiring the skills and fortitude of discriminative discernment is the key to unlocking the power of Patanjali's *Yoga Sutras*. The ego knows what it is: changeable, unconscious, and protective of the self. Othello may be undergoing a spiritual identity crisis, but Iago clearly is not. He blatantly describes his deceptive nature from the get-go by truthfully divulging, "I am not what I am" (1.1).

From a yogic perspective, the term "I am" is often equated with the Divine (or purusha), that which is unchangeable, pure awareness, and all-loving. Once Othello learns the truth, that he has killed his loyal and faithful wife, he regains his soulful Self, his sense of "I am":

When you shall these unlucky deeds relate,
Speak of me as I am. Nothing extenuate,
Nor set down aught in malice. Then must you speak
Of one that loved not wisely, but too well. (5.2)

In this farewell speech, Othello surrenders everything to the truth of who he really is. He drops his mental load. He releases the need for outward reflections of self-image. He no longer needs the ego to make his self-worth dependent on thinking, *I am my victories, I am a husband, I am a revenger, I am anything but who I am, no labels or strings attached.* He simply asks those present to "speak of me as I am." He recognizes his human nature and that he misjudged. But he also reclaims his soul, his true Self, and the awareness that, as a divine being first and foremost, he loved Desdemona wholeheartedly.

Ego Management 101

Through Othello's self-awakening we are given the precious opportunity to learn that we are not our thoughts, our job, our roles as partners, lovers, parents, et cetera, nor our possessions. We are not even our bodies. These perceived layers of our being are all changeable in nature, and our ego knows how uncomfortable it can be to accept their temporal state. In *Yoga Sutras* 1.33–1.39, Patanjali offers seven ways that we can avoid the self-sabotage that arises when the ego throws us off balance and overpowers our true spiritual identity:

○ To preserve openness of heart and calmness of mind, nurture these attitudes:

  ○ Kindness to those who are happy

  ○ Compassion for those who are less fortunate

  ○ Honor for those who embody noble qualities

  ○ Equanimity to those whose actions oppose your values.

○ Slow, easeful exhalations can be used to restore and preserve balance.

○ Or engage the focus on an inspiring object.

○ Or cultivate devotion to the supreme, ever-blissful Light within.

○ Or receive grace from a great soul, who exudes Divine qualities.

○ Or reflect on the peaceful feeling from an experience, a dream, or deep sleep.

○ Or dedicate yourself to anything that elevates and embraces your heart.[5]

Take your pick. When our true nature is obscured by physical, mental, and emotional disturbances, these yogic practices aim to restore and sustain our equanimity.

Yoga is thought-action training, the true grit that Othello and all heroes and heroines, yogis and yoginis alike, need most. Shakespeare's *Othello* reminds us how important it is to put the ego in its rightful place, and yoga philosophy offers us tools for doing so. The practice of asteya infuses a dedication to integrity, a growing awareness of "I am" that the ego knows it is not and finds difficult to compete with. Ego-clinging is the primordial identity theft, but asteya renders such self-inflicted spiritual identity theft obsolete. It promotes not stealing from our unlimited potential.

---

5. Devi, *Secret Power of Yoga*, 75–76.

Putting asteya into practice

By my thirties I was a fervent Bikram yoga student. The practice strengthened my body and sharpened my discipline in a profound way by magnetizing my attention, which was very body-identified at the time. A handful of Bikram teachers cared to know more about a condition I live with called muscular dystrophy (MD) and how the practice helped. But most did not. Bikram and a couple of his teachers asked me to leave or move to the back of their classrooms because I couldn't do the entire practice like everyone else (I kid you not). And yet I kept at it for seven years. All along Bikram was right about that one primary yogic teaching: "Don't let me (meaning him or anyone or anything else, I presume) take your peace away." The message hadn't sunk in yet. The ego had its hold on me.

Even though I had a passionate practice, I held onto the disparaging thought that I could never be a yoga teacher. No way, not with MD. I played the same self-limiting line, like a record player hitting a scratched groove, over and over. My mind was disabled with thinking, *I am limited by disease.*

I shifted to less extreme forms of hot yoga, yin yoga and some power vinyasa. These practices added important variations, life-affirming philosophies, and greater insights into anatomy, including the human energy systems. My life positively transformed. My yogic perspective widened. Looking like everyone else was no longer the goal of my practice; being me was. I also began to understand what was possible in my life: namely, anything I put my mind to—okay, maybe not flying!—but certainly becoming a yoga teacher with or without MD. At age thirty-eight, I trained and taught my first class. Three years later, my husband and I opened the first of three yoga studios in New Zealand, where we eventually led yoga teacher trainings for nearly a decade. MD was never the issue.

It would be too cavalier to say it pays to simply tell the ego to shut up sometimes, although that's true. Shakespeare's plays and yoga teach us it's more than that: activating one's truth takes courage, patience, practice, and, above all, faith. Looking back, all the unnecessary self-sabotaging seems so obvious. The potential for my highest good was there all along. And I imagine that is exactly how Othello must have felt when Iago's treacherous schemes were finally revealed. It was all so obvious, so devastatingly obvious.

The ego is a tricky thing, and self-awareness is often hard-won. As we watch Othello succumb to the seductive allure of the ego, we cringe. We squirm in our seats. We want to warn him, "Don't believe Iago! Put the pillow down! *Turn on* the light! You know the truth, trust it!" But, alas, he does the unthinkable deed: he "puts out the light" every time. Perhaps Shakespeare knew that our empathic response has the potential to trigger a closer look at our own relationship with the ego and how we confront the Iagos in our minds and in our world. Perhaps his play lives on in the hope that we, too, will stop stealing from our vast potential and well-being as individuals and as a society. That "I am" is who we truly are.

CHAPTER 9
The Virtue of Asteya in Shakespeare

To be generous,
guiltless and of free disposition
—Twelfth Night 1.5

Generosity is a positive way of saying nonstealing, and a virtue to which anyone can and should practice, according to the yama of asteya.

In Shakespeare's age, however, "generosity" had a different connotation. As a noun, the word referred to nobility or aristocracy. And the playwright uses the word only once, in the first act of *Coriolanus*: "to break the heart of generosity." Ironically, it's a turbulent opening scene in which generosity as we know it today and in yoga philosophy is lacking. Political unrest is brewing as the people cry for food from the generosity, those in power who have locked up the corn and grain supplies. As an adjective, "generous" likewise implied well-bred or mannerly back then. In Olivia's line "to be generous, / guiltless and of free disposition" (*Twelfth Night* 1.5), "free disposition" is closer to today's use of the word, while "generous" means well mannered. You get the point: the word "generosity" has a rich etymological past; it was a concept reserved for those of high birth until about the seventeenth century.

That said, Shakespearean characters from of all walks of life demonstrate the evolution of the word as we know it today by giving selflessly of their time and resources. Their noble, spirited actions are without thought of remuneration and further our appreciation of Shakespeare's yogic wisdom exemplifying asteya.

Here are just a few examples:

The Winter's Tale shows us the kind Old Shepherd (that's his full name), who finds an abandoned newborn in the Bohemian "desert." "I'll take it up for / pity," he good-naturedly decides, and he raises the "pretty barne" as his own daughter.

In *The Tempest*, Prospero describes Gonzalo's care and concern for their safety in exile to his inquisitive, now-teenage daughter Miranda:

> Some food we had and some fresh water that
> A noble Neapolitan, Gonzalo,
> Out of his charity, being then appointed
> Master of this design, did give us, with
> Rich garments, linens, stuffs and necessaries,
> Which since have steaded much. (*The Tempest* 1.2)

In the same play, Prospero surrenders his life's work—raising Miranda and practicing his potent arts. The magician vows to break his staff and drown his book and to return to Milan so that Miranda may have the future she deserves by marrying Ferdinand.

Duke Senior in *As You Like It* lives exiled in the forest of Arden. Although he admits he's seen better days, he readily shares his meager table with travelers in need. He warmly welcomes them:

> And therefore sit you down in gentleness,
> And take upon command what help we have
> That to your wanting may be minist'red. (*As You Like It* 2.7)

Antonio in *The Merchant of Venice* is a wealthy ship merchant who goes the distance for his dear friend Bassanio by bankrolling his mission to wed the fair Portia. Antonio's generosity is especially poignant in light of textual references indicating that he enjoys Bassanio's companionship himself and because his financial support of Bassanio's amorous endeavor literally puts his own life on the line.

Some folks may contend these are not perfect examples of largesse. The Old Shepherd, for example, finds gold lining the baby basket; Miranda's political gain is a type of return on Prospero's personal divestment; and Antonio may seek Bassanio's everlasting admiration. But any such reciprocation is a perfectly natural by-product of generosity, according to Patanjali. In *Yoga Sutra* 2.37, the sage foresees material and spiritual prosperity bestowed on those abiding in asteya. Ironically, it's when one gives with a pure heart that treasures present themselves. And, as in the case of all five characters mentioned above, in due time, each flourishes in some way from his or her magnanimous actions.

Generating generosity

Current sociological studies verify Patanjali's unshakable truth and Shakespeare's themes illuminate the paradox of generosity. The Science of Generosity Initiative[1] at the College of Notre Dame (Indiana) explores what's going on behind generous behavior and then educates others about their interdisciplinary findings. The Science of Generosity's modern definition of "generosity"—"the virtue of giving good things to others freely and abundantly"—aligns with the ancient wisdom of asteya. It is an essential human virtue to which anyone can aspire, not just those born to a specific class. And it has the potential to make a world-changing, positive difference. Christian Smith and Hilary Davidson's book, *The Paradox of Generosity: Giving We Receive, Grasping We Lose*, further reveals how a regular and consistent practice of generosity equates to a happy, healthier life. Generosity as a way of being gives us a greater purpose. It can be expressed in a creative variety of ways, not just financially, and in the process

---

1. Read more about the initiative at http://generosityresearch.nd.edu/more-about-the-initiative/what-is-generosity/.

connects us to a higher standard of living. Science is catching up with yoga's age-old wisdom.

Generosity is a healthy response to life. But beyond the random act of kindness, how often do we raise our own bar on the practice? Do we, like the Old Shepherd, help shelter those abandoned with donations of food or clothing? Does the plight of people exiled from their homeland or shunned from their families in the name of religion or politics move us to voice our concern and give from the comfort of our secure and well-stocked homes, as Gonzalo examples? As parents, guardians, and elders, do we contribute to the growth and welfare of the next generation, as Prospero demonstrates? Are we inspired by the Duke Senior to likewise assist a traveler in need? And are we, like Antonio, supportive of others' goals and adventures even if that means they may leave us? These are just some of the Bard's proffered opportunities for reflecting and elevating our practice of asteya.

Start where you are

I ask myself these questions: As a yoga teacher, am I giving my best efforts to my students, or am I on cruise control? As a yoga student, do I willingly contribute my energy and resources to benefit the group or studio environment, or do I begrudge my payments and responsibilities? These are simple but powerful questions. And the answers speak volumes on my current level of belief in abundance mentality, the energetic foundation of asteya.

For me as a yoga teacher, preparation and presence are required. These efforts take time and a willingness to set aside personal concerns for a luminous and purposeful collective learning experience. Knowing the dedication and generosity of resources great teachers give, I am always grateful for instructors who consistently bring vigor and fresh ideas to their classes. Their passion for the practice simultaneously instructs and inspires.

As a studio owner for many years, I am likewise deeply moved by students who take it upon themselves to add to the welfare of their learning environment. To our studio, several students brought fresh-picked garden flowers. Others brought their friends who became new regulars.

One practitioner made it her habit to refill the water bottles used for rinsing the mats after class. When I got wind of what she was doing, I said, "You're our guest here. I appreciate your filling the spray bottles, but that's not necessary."

"Oh, it's my joy," she quickly interjected. "I consider it my gift to the studio, my dharma [dharma means 'one's duty and nature']." This woman clearly understood asteya, not to mention the virtue and power of service (*seva*).

I will also never forget the man who insisted on paying for an unlimited month pass even after I suggested to him a ten-card would make the most financial sense based on his attendance. Frankly and intelligently, he responded, "This is my practice and I choose to honor it in this way." I signed him up for another month, extending my deepest gratitude for his contribution and his liberal attitude.

Off the mat and into the world

Generosity expands our focus. There is an important shift from "Me to We" that has both self-reflexive and communal advantages. In *The Art of Happiness in a Troubled World*, the Dalai Lama presents insights on the importance of this shift. He wisely suggests cultivating awareness of our connectedness through a willingness to reach beyond our comfort zones, beyond our fences, beyond our perceptions that isolate us from one another. His words struck a chord in me. Nine months had passed since my husband and I had moved into our new neighborhood, and I still hadn't reached over the fence or ventured beyond a smile and the wave of a hand when passing neighbors. Sure, I had thought about it, plenty of times, but, like a growing number of Westerners, the Dalai Lama points out, I had done nothing in terms of actually reaching out. The Dalai Lama was talking to me. His perceptiveness inspired me to act and, to be perfectly honest, practice what I preach.

And so, I reached out: I baked some cookies and arranged them on paper plates, and I enjoyed the process. Then I rang some doorbells.

The reaction was overwhelming. You would have thought I was Gonzalo pulling back the coverings of the stored necessities on the boat and showing the exiled Duke of Milan that the books he prized above his kingdom were safe aboard. The smiles, the gratitude, that "Come on in!" response was the palpable joy of community in the making. The Dalai Lama was right: it is the *willingness* that matters.

As a result of that simple gesture, which could have been anything heartfelt (although the cookies were really good), I was reminded once again of the principle of asteya. A couple of days later, I was invited out for coffee by one neighbor; with another, brief hellos while walking her dog developed into lingering, lovely conversations. Barbecues and invitations to events have become more frequent, and talk of a block party and other community outreach activities grow in earnest.

Looking for ways to grow more generous starts where you are. We need not wait for a Shakespearean drama to rock our world, an abandoned baby to show up at our doorstep, a friend to request a sizable loan, or hungry travelers to cross our path in the woods. These opportunities are all around us, and they are for us to activate our most generous response possible. Volunteering, donating, adding on a bit extra when theaters and nonprofit organizations ask for funding, et cetera, are purposeful actions. They are the positive and proactive reflexes of asteya. And, when performed on a regular basis, they raise our spirits, improve our health, and unify our world. They are the win-win performances on this great stage of life.

Bramacharya

Moderation and Balance

CHAPTER 10
Brahmacharya as Reflected in *Romeo and Juliet*

Ask God for temperance; that's the appliance [remedy] *only*
Which your disease requires.
— The Life of King Henry VIII 1.1

Romeo and Juliet live in a city off kilter. Opposition reigns. Life-changing events, both hostile and passionate, spark quickly. Family feuds rage. Lethal weapons whip out at the slightest provocation. Political decrees are strict and readily ignored. Parents try to fast-forward their children's lives while, behind the scenes, their kids beat them to the punch by taking matters of life and death into their own hands. It's just plain hard to relax with so much extreme in the air. Verona is the perfect setting to witness Shakespeare's yogic teachings on *brahmacharya*, the needful practice of moderation and balance.

A balancing act
Although all the yamas are about how we treat others, the fourth yama, brahmacharya, directs the outward, socially oriented nature of the yamas more inward. There is a growing element of self-discipline associated with the yoga practice of brahmacharya; it requires strength of mind that relies on the previously present-ed three yamas of ahimsa (nonviolence), satya (truthfulness), and asteya (nonstealing). Brahmacharya is also the most highly contested of the yamas, as strict interpretations have defined it

as sexual chastity rather than as a conscious moderation of the expenditure of sexual energy, or any energy for that matter, and directing it toward a higher purpose, like study or prayer or greater overall vitality. Patanjali puts it this way:

> Devoted to living a balanced and moderate life (Brahmacharya), the scope of one's life force becomes boundless. (*Yoga Sutra* 2.38)[1]

Love rollercoaster

Romeo and Juliet are thought to be adolescents; several times throughout the play, Romeo is referred to as a "young" man and Juliet is said to be "of a pretty age," (*Romeo and Juliet* 2.4) not quite fourteen. According to Vedic traditions, they are in the stage of life that, like the yama, is also called brahmacharya, a time when the enormous outburst of sexual energy should be channeled for educational development. If not, a large part of a child's potential will be squandered, making it tougher to harness again later in life. In thoughtful response to Paris's suit to wed Juliet in Act 1, Capulet alludes to the importance of carefully timing his daughter Juliet's marriage:

CAPULET
My child is yet a stranger in the world.
She hath not seen the change of fourteen years.
Let two more summers wither in their pride
Ere we may think her ripe to be a bride.

PARIS
Younger than she are happy mothers made.

CAPULET
And too soon marred are those so early made. (1.2)

---

1. Devi, *Secret Power of Yoga*, 193.

Shakespeare's legendary Seven Ages of Man speech in *As You Like It* picks up on the ancient categorization of life's divided parts and the roles we play. Jacques, who delivers the famous discourse, describes stage three as "the lover, sighing like a furnace, with a woeful ballad made to his mistress' eyebrow" (*As You Like It* 2.7). The star-crossed lovers fall squarely into this category and the sexual chemistry they exude is legendary. *Romeo and Juliet* is a play that continues to appeal to teenagers because it's all about navigating the tempestuous surge of thoughts and feelings that get stirred up in a young lover in the age of brahmacharya.[2]

The basic expression of the life force is sexual energy. And, as yoga is essentially an internal balancing act, mastering our sensual desires, even our most primal ones, is key. Shakespeare purposefully and liberally uses bawdy innuendos and language smacking of sexual import throughout his works because he too understands how vital sex is to the average person's human experience. Sex gets our attention. (Just ask any advertiser or film producer today.) Besides, if Romeo and Juliet had just met for coffee, we'd have no play and no lessons in the necessity of moderation, abstention, and the patience they require, would we?

Checks and imbalances

Romeo and Juliet are the only offspring of Verona's two noble houses, precious jewels to their parents and their community. But in most respects, they are just ordinary kids dealing with ordinary urges. Shakespeare provides each of them with a person to whom they can speak freely and whom they can ask for advice outside the rules and regulations of parents and the strict social

---

2. The issue of consensual sex between minors continues to be debated today. Several US states have "Romeo and Juliet laws" that govern the age of consent. These laws attempt to correct what some courts have deemed overly harsh laws regarding consensual teenage sex.

order. Although the Nurse serves as Juliet's confidante until Act 3 (when she suddenly shifts alliance to Juliet's parents), it is Friar Laurence in whom the lovers most seek safe haven and "good counsel." Critics of Laurence imply that his swift decision to marry Romeo and Juliet is solely political, to unite the feuding households. That observation is certainly valid. Friar Laurence is as human as a character as the rest of the cast and subject to his own imperfections, which more often than not contradict his own sound advice. But the advice he does give is grounded spiritual wisdom nonetheless, wisdom that is needed as much in today's world as it is in Shakespeare's Verona.

Fabio Toblini,[3] the costume designer for the Broadway production of *Romeo and Juliet* (2013), describes Friar Laurence as "a hermit who lives removed from church politics, an independent thinker, and a spiritual human being who wants what's best for the teens, even if that means working in a way that gets around the law."[4] Contemporary yet "timeless," Toblini's costuming of the friar reflects what he believes the hermit spiritualist represents most: neutrality. Toblini attired the actor playing Friar Laurence (Brent Carver) in a hooded tunic shirt with loose, flowing pants, handcrafted sandals, and a shoulder-slung canvas tote bag, all in earthy hues of blue and beige—like a kind of new-age hippy, and a look strikingly similar to what yoga clothing shops stock for men today. Directorial shifts furthered the friar's costuming and role as latent peacemaker: positioned next to caged doves, Friar Laurence takes on the play's opening prologue flashing the modern-day hand gesture for peace on the first word, "Two." And, at its sorrowful ending, he tolls a large church bell signaling sad, spiritual release.[5] Ultimately, however, as in any production

---

3. http://fabiotoblini.com.
4. Fabio Toblini, interview with author, 11 July 2014.
5. https://www.youtube.com/watch?v=HWPy584__gM.

and its interpretation of Friar Laurence, it's Shakespeare's lines that fill the role, and so much of the friar's dialogue conveys the principles of brahmacharya.

Enter Romeo

Even before we first see Romeo, we know he walks the hills pining for Rosaline, a chaste young woman. This doting affection will be so brief we'll never see her onstage. (The rare exception being Franco Zeffirelli's 1968 film version, in which a brilliant visual reference to Rosaline dancing reveals Juliet as Rosaline spins away. Romeo looks on, spontaneously dropping his infatuation for Rosaline and falling in love at first sight with Juliet. He's hooked.) By Act 2, Romeo bursts into the friar's cell, insisting the friar marry him to "the fair daughter of rich Capulet."

> When and where and how
> We met, we wooed and made exchange of vow,
> I'll tell thee as we pass, but this I pray:
> That thou consent to marry us today. (*Romeo and Juliet* 2.3)

As an audience, we often laugh.

And we worry. Romeo's youthful impetuousness may be charming but it also bodes a dangerous downfall. We know because we have witnessed this type of reckless, desiring behavior and its effects before: in ourselves and our kids, in our colleagues, even in our political and social leaders. But being human doesn't excuse or help our lives in these situations; exercising a healthy dose of restraint to temper our course does.

Balancing Romeo's inherent lack of temperance, Friar Laurence offers repeated counsel on moderation, patience, and abstinence, all elements of brahmacharya. For example, a piece of advice Romeo gets from Friar Laurence on the importance of pacing serves us as well as it does him:

ROMEO
O, let us hence; I stand on sudden haste.

FRIAR LAURENCE
Wisely and slow; they stumble that run fast. (2.3)[6]

Shakespeare understands the necessity of pacing ourselves in a world that loves speed. Heeding the advice to contemplate, to examine our impulses before acting, brings clarity to our life purpose and our yoga practice. Like Romeo, the "young waverer," as the friar calls him, we are reminded to consciously create a life that does not keep us running after our ever-changing desires.

Soon again, the friar instructs Romeo on obtaining long-lasting love: "love moderately; long love doth so" (2.6)—again, brahmacharya in poetic verse, plain and simple. Most people want a happy, healthy life, but without moderation we fritter away our time, energy, and resources, compromising that which we often hold most dear. Overeating, overworking, compulsive shopping, over- or undersleeping, satiating every sexual desire, or, conversely, unreasonably repressing our natural urges, even practicing yoga asana without regard to the physical ebb and flow of our bodies, puts us squarely in Romeo's court. We, too, are the friar's loving pupils and have everything to gain by heeding his guidance.

A happy medium in all things is needed if we are to enjoy life fully. But, like Romeo and Juliet, many of us live in a time and place of excess and extreme. Maintaining a balanced lifestyle becomes a conscious, everyday yogic practice that, although seemingly challenging, is worthy of directed efforts to simplify our lives. For, as Indian philosopher Jiddu Krishnamurti observes, "It is no measure of health to be well adjusted to a profoundly sick society."[7]

---

6. In Zeffirelli's film adaptation, adhering to traditional interpretations, ironically Friar Laurence himself trips on a church cobblestone directly after speaking this line.

7. http://www.wildmind.org/blogs/quote-of-the-month/krishnamurti-measure-of-health

Patience, you must have

Romeo's reactivity is tenacious. Patience and clearheadedness in times of emotional upheaval are not one of his strong suits. When banished from Verona for killing Tybalt (Juliet's cousin), Friar Laurence restores Romeo's equilibrium by broadening his fixated, narrow focus on banishment with the promise of a future reunited with his wife, Juliet: "Be patient for the world is broad and wide" (3.3).

Romeo's rashness, however, does not allow for other explanations of the rumor of Juliet's "death," and when the friar is not present to help him think things through, he reverts back to his brooding, impatient self. Brahmacharya requires an element of self-disciplined patience that Romeo lacks, a mindfulness that considers the benefits of refraining from jumping to conclusions, immediately striking back, or satiating every sensual longing as soon as possible. Even Juliet, very early on anyway, chides his sexual impatience and desiring nature:

> I have no joy of this contract tonight.
> It is too rash, too unadvised, too sudden,
> Too like the lightning which doth cease to be
> Ere one can say it lightens. (2.1)

Romeo is surrounded by people who want what's best for him; the friar and his closest friends, Benvolio and Mercutio, all strive to balance his mood swings and reactive personality. But, as with us, tempering a changeable constitution is ultimately personal work requiring spiritual maturity.

I often quote Friar Laurence in my yin yoga classes. While the body strengthens and lengthens, there is ample time to train the mind with some of the Bard's take on what brahmacharya as a mindfulness practice is all about. Our limited perception of what we think life offers in any given moment makes us impatient.

Immediate gratification can supersede considered action. In yoga postures (asana), we may want to make our move before the time is ripe to do so. We prefer to be done with this or that posture or the class itself and return to the outward satisfactions of our known and comfortable world. This impatience only placates us. Learning to sit with whatever arises in our practice is our practice. Our discomfort gives us the opportunity to examine the motive of our thoughts and desires and see them for the illusions they are. In turn, those very thoughts and desires often release their hold. Clearer insights arise. We can be spiritually directed toward other possible truths. And, as Patanjali promises, we feel a sense of liberation.

Life's ups and downs

From womb to tomb, there are three modes of being that we or any aspect of nature (prakriti) experiences. These three qualities of nature are called the *gunas*: *sattva, rajas,* and *tamas*. Sattva is a state of harmonious balance. For example, it's how you feel when the body gets both proper exercise and sufficient rest. Your physical, mental, and emotional engines purr smoothly. Rajas relates to motion and stimulation; tamas denotes a state of inactivity or rest. We need both rajas and tamas. Rajas fires our engines when we feel sluggish or need to act quickly, and tamas slows us down when we are in overdrive or require sanctuary. By respecting the ebb and flow of our natural rhythms, we live an overall sattvic, or balanced, lifestyle. Naturally occurring fluctuations of the gunas cannot be arrested, nor should they be. Some argue that one state is not better than another. Each of the three states has its purpose. *Yoga Sutra* 2.18 describes the role of gunas:

> Nature, its three qualities, *sattva, rajas,* and *tamas,* and its
> evolutes, the elements, mind, senses of perception and organs

of action, exist externally to serve the seer, for enjoyment or emancipation.[8]

As humans we are always striving for balance. We are always in motion, even when we think we're standing still. Close your eyes while standing in Mountain Pose (*tadasana*) and you immediately feel the subtle push-pull of gravity, time, and space. Try to empty your mind and within nanoseconds a thought barges in. These experiences remind us that the sway of the gunas affects our physical and mental states until the moment of our spiritual liberation. The more conscious we are of our predominant patterns, the more we can shorten the swing between rajas and tamas and increase our physical health, mental stability, and overall happiness. We recognize that we can rise above them, even if temporarily. However, if a highly rajasic or a predominantly tamasic lifestyle is left unchecked, life becomes a rollercoaster of stressful ups and downs that deplete our energy, inducing depression, disease, and suffering. Romeo and Juliet ride that rollercoaster and Shakespeare structures the play and its language around their dramatic turn of events.

The play opens with a brief, balanced statement, sattvic in nature: "Two households, both alike in dignity, / In fair Verona, we lay our scene" (*Romeo and Juliet* Prologue).

And, as we shall hear in the play itself, equal syllables weight Romeo with Juliet and Montague with Capulet, a device the playwright uses in many of his plays to emphasize an inherent social equality between the characters.

But from the opening lines forward, heavy contrasts in thematic and verbal structure will transform all of Verona, most especially the star-crossed lovers. The first half of the play starts

---

8. Iyengar, *Light on the Yoga Sutras*, 125.

out primarily rajasic, high-spirited and energetic. Many events strike us as a romantic comedy, full of witty play, dancing, and matchmaking. The summer escapades of teens looking for trouble appear to be a natural by-product of the incendiary atmosphere. But Verona's world proves unbalanced at every turn. And, as you listen, you hear lines packed with opposites and extremes. One example is from Tybalt in Act 1, Scene 1: "What, drawn [sword] and talk of peace?" And another, in an aside by Juliet in Act 1, Scene 5: "My only love sprung from my only hate!"

Act 3, Scene 1, positioned midway through the play, marks the fulcrum before the scales must naturally tip. As Mercutio, perhaps the most lively and imaginative character of the play, lies dying, he snarls a parting curse that echoes the first line of the prologue, though in dark reverse, "A plague o' both your houses . . . . Your houses!" After this momentary balance of shared accountability, the play reboots, but now as a tragedy full of destruction and transformation.

Romeo feels the tamasic weight bear down. The fun and games are over. The blush of young love has brought forth the responsibilities of marriage, and carefree days are replaced with the serious repercussions of murder. The teens must grow up overnight, choosing self-directed actions over parental dictates. Deep sleep, dark choices, and death are now the introspective, cooling elements that a play turned upside down leaves in its gloomy, glorious wake.

The passion problem

When it comes to passion, most people think of blissful, adrenaline-riddled highs. Shakespeare's *Romeo and Juliet* or perhaps his later work *Antony and Cleopatra* comes to mind close behind. An awareness of the gunas illuminates Shakespeare's knowledge of passion's beauty and also of its ultimately unsustainable extreme.

Suffering is a less-remembered definition of passion. And many forget that the flip side of following one's bliss is the work it takes to manifest that bliss. Passion as a human longing produces magnificence, inspires amazing dedication, and generates enormous sacrifice. Passion fuels the arts, technological advancements, world exploration, even our spiritual practices. And although passion for anything or anyone moves us to great heights, we suffer if our focus and purpose do not honor the principle of brahmacharya. Stress-related illnesses, cortisol-fueled work environments, and increasingly sedentary lifestyles are maladaptive by-products when a society loses touch with the natural and necessary rhythms of nature. Yoga aims to regulate us so that earning an income or following our heart's desire does not take precedence over living a well-rounded life.

Friar Laurence and Patanjali are right to teach us moderation. Otherwise, as Shakespeare's heroes so clearly demonstrate, our bodies and minds, both part of the natural world, do it for us. Brahmacharya advises a middle way that makes us ultimately more productive and more vibrant beings. A good way to remember this yama is to think of life as a carpenter's level, for which the aim is to keep the bubble in between the lines. Some may scoff at that thought as being safe or boring. But knowing that a recurrent rise and fall of the gunas is part of balancing that level spices life with purpose and variation while ensuring sufficient time to reflect and restore the life force.

How we cope and grow as a result of life's ups and downs reflects the degree to which brahmacharya is a conscious part of our practice. Advancing in yoga is not about doing more complicated postures; it's about becoming curious as to how the body works best. After a day at the computer, a rajasic yoga asana practice (like power vinyasa) balances out sitting all day. In hot weather, a restorative tamasic practice (like yin yoga) may be a better choice.

Sex, drugs, and rock and roll have their time and place, but without regular cleansing practices such as yoga, meditation, and trust in the natural remedy of a balanced lifestyle, we quickly drain our life force, not to mention our sex appeal. Our bodies and minds are not automated machines. They are organic organisms, forever changing. Seasonal, daily, sometimes hourly, monitoring and regular fine-tuning are required. What needs to happen to center the bubble in the level varies for each of us. And this process is called yoga, a process of regaining wholeness and balance. Along the path of that discovery there will be many teachers, gurus, and guides. Romeo and Juliet had Friar Laurence. He is a character through whom Shakespeare life-coaches not only the world's most famous adolescents, but us too. The question is: Are we heeding his yogic advice regarding brahmacharya?

CHAPTER 11

Brahmacharya as Reflected in *Henry IV, Part 1*; *Henry IV, Part 2*; and *Henry V*

If all the year were playing holidays,
To sport would be as tedious as to work
—Henry IV, Part 1 1.2

The importance of brahmacharya (moderation and balance) naturally points us to one of Shakespeare's most beloved comic characters, a bon vivant named Sir John Falstaff. This witty, fat old knight makes audiences laugh with his excesses in every regard: feasting, whoring, drinking, lying, purse pinching, even loud snoring. His general disregard for moderation of any sort makes for highly entertaining theater, and yet underneath the slapstick and pointed socio-political humor, his character educates. Audiences adore him for fully embracing human creature comforts, but I wouldn't say they necessarily admire or aspire to his lifestyle. Falstaff pays a high price for his choices. And the painful repercussions of those choices are not lost on his friend (who happens to be the heir apparent, Prince Henry), nor on us.

Paying the price

A urine sample reveals that Falstaff "might have more diseases than he knew for," including the "gout" and not one, but several forms of syphilis (*Henry IV, Part 2* 1.2). Ultimately, he is rightly nicknamed "Monsieur Remorse." Prince Henry (also known as

Hal) taunts him, referring to him as "that reverend vice, that grey iniquity, that father ruffian, that vanity in years" (*Henry IV, Part 1* 3.2). And yet we, like Hal, can't help but love Falstaff for his "suchness"—his unabashedly full sense of who he thinks he is, which in his case appears to be solely a merry Lord of Misrule, and what makes him tick. Falstaff doesn't take worldly concerns as dramatic emergencies. He rolls between the royal court and the Boar's Head Tavern with ease, and no one is above a dose of his superb ability to misdirect the truth. Falstaff even takes Hal's ongoing fat jokes without bitterness or self-pity, perhaps because underneath the blubber and buckram lies a soul who would readily agree with Macbeth's conclusion, that life is "a tale / told by an idiot, full of sound and fury / Signifying nothing" (*Macbeth* 5.5), so why take it all—war, work, honor, proper care of the body—so seriously? Falstaff balances out anyone who is need of a good laugh, even if it's at his own expense. By making a mockery of everything, however, Falstaff also injects the world with a social disorder and rebellion that becomes as claustrophobic as the politics he abhors. Prince Hal comments that a life of total debauchery also grows downright boring after a while: "If all the year were playing holidays, / To sport would be as tedious as to work" (*Henry IV, Part 1* 1.2).

Deep down, Falstaff, like many of us, longs for greater balance in life. Given the chance of advancement, even Falstaff admits going on a diet and giving up drinking sack (sherry) would do him good:

> He that rewards
> me, God reward him. If I do grow great, I'll grow
> less, for I'll purge and leave sack and live cleanly as
> a nobleman should do. (5.4)

But wishful thinking for the perfect conditions to begin choosing brahmacharya as a lifestyle will never bring them about.

Festivals and holidays purposefully interrupt the routines of every culture. Celebrating the gifts of the season lifts our spirits while reminding us of traditions designed to unify and elevate our souls. However, these same events can easily drain our energy and our bank accounts if not managed with spiritual care. As a yoga studio owner, I often spied a layer of weariness in students as they signed in for class during the holiday season. And you could always count on an increase in new students and returning students after the first of the year or as spring arrived. After the indulgences associated with holidays or the heavier meals and long resting phase of winter, it is the practice of brahmacharya that propels people into detox mode, a fresh start, and the promise of better health.

Brahmacharya is a natural choice if we are listening to our bodies. Letting go, indulging, and dropping our practice is perfectly healthy for a short spell every now and then, but when a break is prolonged for weeks, months, or years, the chance for depression, illness, and financial ruin runs high. Falstaff's demise is an example.

In the final act of *Henry IV, Part 2*, Hal, now the newly crowned King Henry V, banishes his former tavern buddy until he cleans up his act. The royal command "not to come near our person by ten mile" (*Henry IV, Part 2* 5.5) comes as a complete and utter blow to Falstaff (and to many audience members), and the heartrending disappointment has a dire emotional and physical effect on Falstaff. Not only has he lost his best friend and the chance of advancement that such an alliance might have guaranteed, he is also 1000 pounds in debt (if not more) and riddled with disease. In the Shakespeare's Globe production of *Henry IV, Part 2* (London, 2010), Roger Allam's award-winning portrayal of Falstaff captures the devastating effect Hal's dramatic, though subtly forewarned, decree of banishment has on Falstaff's mind-body connection. Allam's Falstaff, one who has nimbly averted danger and duty and eaten and entertained himself through two plays, suddenly hunches over, his hands shaking with shock and grief. Instantaneously, he shows signs of aging and ill health. In this defining "marker event," Allam's contrast in body language speaks volumes on yoga philosophy, specifically wisdom often attributed to the Upanishads, one of the sources for Patanjali's *Yoga Sutras*:

> Watch your thoughts; they become words.
> Watch your words; they become actions.
> Watch your actions; they become habits.
> Watch your habits; they become your character.
> Watch your character; it becomes your destiny.

Falstaff never recovers. A lifetime of intemperate choices has caught up with him. As *Henry V* begins, he dies, offstage, with complications related to some sexually transmitted disease and brokenhearted. His tavern hostess, Mistress Quickly, laments, "The king has killed his heart" (*Henry V* 2.1).

Or has he? Although Falstaff has served as a surrogate father to the prince, offering the young swag a time and place to release the pressures of court as he navigates his rise to power, he, like all of us, can't escape the yogic notion that our biography becomes our biology.[1] That the choices we make shape our outcome. That someone can love us but consciously choose not to facilitate our negative patterns of behavior at some point. That eventually tough love like King Henry V's, karma, or nature itself eventually evens out our imbalances. The ancient wisdom of brahmacharya and the relationship between Falstaff and Hal teach us to embrace all

---

1. Caroline Myss, *Anatomy of the Spirit: The Seven Stages of Power and Healing* (New York: Three Rivers Press, 1996), 34, 40–43, 45, 58.

aspects of life, not just the ones we like, as opportunities to learn, transform, and prosper with less suffering.

Bodybuilding

Falstaff's turbocharged carousing is not the only cautionary tale about the importance of moderation and balance in the first two plays in which he appears, *Henry IV, Part 1* and *Henry IV, Part 2*.[2] Each of the four main characters in *Henry IV, Part 1*—Henry IV, Falstaff, Hotspur and Hal—demonstrate imbalances associated with his character, or humor, as it was called in Elizabethan medicinal circles. (The word "humor" did not take on its current meaning until the 17th century.)

The four humors—melancholy, phlegmatic, choleric, and sanguine—correspond to the circular rhythms of the elements, the seasons, and the time of the day, in turn affecting the blood, organs, physical attributes, and behavorial tendencies. Similar to the Ayurvedic wisdom of the three *doshas*, one humor is not necessarily better than another. "Every humour hath his adjunct pleasure, / Wherein it finds a joy above the rest," Shakespeare penned for Sonnet 91.[3] Perhaps for this reason, in *Henry IV, Part 1*, the playwright gives roughly equal lines to melancholy Henry IV (338), phlegmatic Falstaff (542), choleric Hotspur (538), and sanguine Prince Henry (514).[4] In this play (and moving into *Henry IV, Part 2* and *Henry V*, as well), the marked contrast between the four humors not only colors the wording of the play, it underpins the four main characters' motives. Their humoral excesses and deficiencies drive the action. Humorism becomes another yoga

---

2. Falstaff later returns to the stage by popular demand in *The Merry Wives of Windsor*.
3. http://theshakespeareblog.com/2014/02/sadness-and-the-four-humours-in-shakespeare/
4. http://scholarcommons.usf.edu/cgi/viewcontent.cgi?article=1229&context=etd; William Shakespeare, *King Henry IV, Part 1*, ed. David Scott Karstan (London: Thomas Learning, 2002).

lesson in brahmacharya on the ways the health of the microcosm affects the health of the macrocosm. Shakespeare establishes a mind-body plot that simultaneously weaves humor health, or lack thereof, with public events beginning with the opening lines of *Henry IV, Part 1*. A troubled, melancholy king proclaims:

> So shaken as we are, so wan with care,
> Find we a time for frighted peace to pant
> And breathe short-winded accents of new broils
> To be commenced in strands afar remote. (*King Henry IV, Part 1* 1.1)

As Henry IV's health fails, unrest in his kingdom grows. As Prince Henry tempers his humor, England gains political stability. Such humor-oriented comparisons will carry throughout the entire trilogy.

"A yogi never forgets health must begin with the body," yoga master B.K.S. Iyengar states.[5] From there, yoga practices draw the attention inward, developing more subtle layers of being to awaken consciousness. With practice, the true Self presides, calmly and with clear-seeing. Learning how the body works best in response to breath work (pranayama) and conscious movement (asana) is a large part of beginning a yoga practice. So too with Shakespeare's yoga. Understanding qualities of a particular constitution plays a large role in successfully preventing and healing diseases, growing in spiritual maturity, and successfully reaping the practical benefits of brahmacharya.

It takes all types

Belief in the humors and their impact on human well-being laces many of Shakespeare's plays, but the dynamic interplay of the

---

5. B. K. S. Iyengar, *Light on Life: The Yoga Journey to Wholeness, Inner Peace, and Ultimate Freedom* (Emmaus, PA: Rodale, 2005), 23.

humors is particularly instructive in *Henry IV, Part 1* and *Part 2*. A balance must be struck, internally and externally.

Representing melancholy is the plays' title character. King Henry IV is losing sleep over his wayward son, Prince Henry, and feels Hal's loose behavior is a punishment for murdering Richard II, from whom he literally took the crown. Familial concerns, compounded with fears of disloyalty, are stressing him out and making him quite sick. Like Shakespeare's other famous melancholy personalities, Hamlet and Jacques (from *As You Like It*), King Henry IV tends to be intelligent, introspective, and, given the opportunity, a bit long-winded and given to fits. King Henry IV's humoral traits motivate his dialogue in court and power up some rather lengthy father-son talks through which Hal must sit and suffer his father's one-sided point of view of what it means to be a prince:

> Could such inordinate and low desires,
> Such poor, such bare, such lewd, such mean attempts,
> Such barren pleasures, rude society
> As thou art matched withal, and grafted to,
> Accompany the greatness of thy blood,
> And hold their level with thy princely heart? (3.2)

It's no wonder Hal turns to Falstaff for some levity. His father continually and quite thoroughly reminds him of life's responsibilities; Falstaff's conversations are loaded with witty play and the pursuit of life's pleasures. Many humorists consider Sir John Falstaff to be phlegmatic: prone to slothful, cowardly behavior, and corpulent. Shakespeare obviously creates a character who fits the bill, though others argue he also exhibits signs of sanguinity—as he is lively, prone to laughter, and red-cheeked, albeit due to an excess of liquor (water), which is a phlegmatic trait.[6] The

---

6. And that theory is entirely plausible, given that many constitutions are blended humors (or doshas).

phlegmatic humor is associated with the hours of 3 pm to 9 pm, the time Falstaff says he was born: "I was born about three of the clock in the afternoon, / with a white head and something a round belly" (*Henry IV, Part 2* 1.2). Prince Henry jests that it's also the time Falstaff habitually starts his day:

> Thou art so fat-witted, with drinking of old sack
> and unbuttoning thee after supper and sleeping upon
> benches after noon, that thou hast forgotten to
> demand that truly which thou wouldst truly know.
> (*Henry IV, Part 1* 1.2)

Falstaff's utter lack of ambition, except for getting his hands on more money and sack, juxtaposes Henry IV's humoral motives in reverse. Staged between these two men, Hal keenly observes both his imbalanced melancholy father and excessive phlegmatic father figure, taking mental notes. The former triggers self-rejection; the latter, self-loathing. Until he can integrate the two humors into an understanding of who he is, Hal remains fragmented.

And then there's Hotspur, known more formally in court as Harry Percy. As a humor archetype, he represents choleric: summer, ambition, a ruling nature, and quick thinking. Here we see a brave young man who has seen blood and battle and lives solely to work. Just ask his wife. He's also making Hal look ever more the slacker for most of *Henry IV, Part 1*. As his name indicates, though, Hotspur is also fiery, highly impatient, and unwilling to hear any reasoning but his own. When told that King Henry IV is onto his plan to usurp the throne and to reconsider, he responds straightaway, "I am on fire!" (*Henry IV, Part 1* 4.1). Choleric types, like the Nike athletic slogan, are all about "Just do it." Now, Hotspur's driving ambition to "pluck bright honor from the pale-faced moon" (1.3) may be admirable, even justifiable, but his timing is off. An imbalanced choleric temperament leads to impulsivity and anger and, in Hotspur's case, to his quick demise. His flame extinguishes in Act 5 of *Henry IV, Part 1*.

As mentioned previously, as *Henry IV, Part 1* opens, the bad-boy prince, Hal, thoroughly enjoys tavern hopping with Falstaff and revels in their antics (as much we do). But, all along, he knows avoiding his duties at court and a life of constant partying are not a good long-term career option. Falstaff claims Hal has inherited his father's "cold blood," but—all thanks to drinking a good amount of sherry with him—"he [Hal] is become very hot and valiant" (*Henry IV, Part 2* 4.3). Although no one would take Falstaff's medical analysis of the humors as reliable, the point is this: Hal's predominant humor grows increasingly temperate. He is not his father; he is not another Falstaff in the making; nor is his leadership destined to copy Hotspur's old-world domination style. As the hero, Prince Henry is cast as sanguine. Balanced sanguine types exude the optimism of spring and a generosity of spirit. Imbalanced, they are prone to irresponsibility. As yogis, what we see in Prince Henry is a growing, conscious effort to balance his humor. To feel comfortable with who he is as a human being and with his dharma. For most of us, Hal included, this is slow work that takes time.

Through an interplay of the four humors, Shakespeare's yoga incites our curiosity yet again: Where do I see a reflection of myself in the humors? What lifestyle choices best balance my constitution? What yoga practices would help? What foods, climates, and occupations suit me? How can a conscious effort to balance my mind-body connection positively affect others? Seeking the answers to these questions is the practice of brahmacharya. From a yogic viewpoint, caring for the self is not a matter of "shoulds." It's a process of compassionate curiosity that gradually reveals our authenticity. It's about looking in the mirror, really looking, and lovingly embracing a visceral reconnection to the unique needs of the body and mind. As conscious observers of the play, we pause and reflect.

Similar to the four humors, Eastern approaches to healing, such as yoga, Ayurveda, and Traditional Chinese Medicine (TCM), view the cells that make up our tissues, organs, and skin as energy. Any disease, or dis-ease, is therefore an energetic imbalance that is proactively addressed from the inside out, slowly and naturally. These healing methods understand the patterns of nature and recognize that the body is its own ecosystem. The use of appropriate diet, herbs, acupuncture, cupping, massage, or some combination of these is based on the varying patterns for each person's constitution. While the disease processes may not be fully reversed, they can often be slowed, with symptoms reducing in severity. I cannot overemphasize the tremendous benefits I have received by utilizing such holistic treatments. They strengthen my inner well-being, which better fuels the energy for my structural needs, including my asana practice.

Being the change

Throughout the trilogy in which he stars, Prince Henry refines his capacity for equanimity in himself and, in turn, for England. He is, like any yogi, on the quest for his true Self. He strives to align the subtle layers of his being in order to shine more gloriously—not just to pad his ego, but in order to serve as a better king. Likewise, the yamas are choices that improve life and reduce suffering for others, and will naturally reflect in our own well-being too.

In *Henry IV, Part 1*, the prince plans to socially redeem himself by showing the world that he can change his behavior and the company he keeps. That he can, as he promises his disgruntled father, the king, "be more myself" (*Henry IV, Part 1* 3.2). Although somewhat calculated, Hal's intended self-transformation reminds us that we too have the potential to rebalance our lives and that, despite our own forms of intemperance, change is possible, not to mention inspiring to others.

PRINCE HENRY
So when this loose behavior I throw off,
And pay the debt I never promisèd,
By how much better than my word I am,
By so much shall I falsify men's hopes;
And, like bright metal on a sullen ground,
My reformation, glitt'ring o'er my fault,
Shall show more goodly and attract more eyes
Than that which hath no foil to set it off. (1.2)

When Prince Henry kills Hotspur in battle, he temporarily regains emotional ground with his father. That said, yoga tells us transformation is a process. Fits and starts are to be expected. Self-discipline (the niyama of tapas) and self-study (the niyama of svadhyaya) correspond to brahmacharya, as these personal observances are essential to moving us toward a balance of mind and body despite inevitable setbacks.

Hal returns to Eastcheap for another round of revelry with Falstaff in *Henry IV, Part 2*. His archetypal quest to gracefully inhabit both the ordinary world of "every Jack" and the royal court is not yet complete. His shadow side is not yet fully integrated. His dharma looms in the near future, but until the prince's humor is balanced, his character remains disjointed. Likewise, England.

Healing lessons

Toward the close of *Henry IV, Part 2*, Hal, thinking his father has taken his last breath (though he hasn't—oops!), tries on the crown and momentarily leaves the room with it. I like to think it is to see an outward vision of his true Self in a mirror and privately attempt to internalize that which he has avoided and with which he is slowly coming to terms. But something is missing, and Shakespeare makes that readily known. When the king momentarily revives and discovers that his son has prematurely taken his crown, only forgiveness and blessings—ahimsa, the essential element of all yamas—make personal integration possible for both father and son. The inner wars raging within them come to a ceasefire. Their humors, after two full-length plays, finally begin to balance, and hope is restored both personally and politically.

The prolonged effects of imbalanced humors, disease, and dying themes weigh heavily in *Henry IV, Part 2*. Because Hal is the only character consciously working to temper his character, he alone survives to the end of the trilogy. The four humors in Shakespeare's plays encourage us to see any disease as an opportunity for self-inquiry. Is there a symbolic story at a higher level of consciousness that underpins our disease? When we take the time to be with this question, an empowering healing process activates within us. We scan our hearts and minds for unresolved issues or related life events with a similar emotional punch. Accepting our insights as our own cherry-picked life lesson, we can then—here's the best part!—let the dis-ease go. This choice, to love and learn from what is, lightens our darkest days. It leads to forgiveness and true healing, that of our spirit. This is brave and conscious work. And although this self-reflective process doesn't guarantee remission or reversal, it does offer something we often practice yoga for in the first place: a soulful peace. Our consciousness stretches its parameters to include any experience as an acceptable expression of life and self-growth.

Patanjali's *Yoga Sutras* tell us that brahmacharya increases the life force. Hal not only becomes Henry V, he becomes the change he (along with his late father) wants to see for England. Comfortable in his skin, his humor better balanced through moderation, a successful leader emerges, one who is as effective in court as he is on the battlefield fighting alongside ordinary men who achieve extraordinary victory. His life force increasingly influences and inspires others. Shortly before the Battle of Agincourt, the best of his persuasive sanguine energy emanates in his famous St. Crispin's Day speech. He creates a "band of brothers" and wins the day. His journey highlights the promise of brahmacharya, a life that unites as it keeps turning toward insight and balance. He is our yoga lesson in the powerful benefits of practicing brahmacharya.

CHAPTER 12

Brahmacharya as Reflected in *As You Like It* and *A Midsummer Night's Dream*

And this our life, exempt from public haunt,
Finds tongues in trees, books in the running brooks,
Sermons in stones, and good in everything.
—*As You Like It* 2.1

There is a less-remembered definition of brahmacharya that Shakespeare's yoga exemplifies. The yama brahmacharya literally refers to living a life in which you are always aware of Divinity, of the Supreme Intelligence.

Breaking down the word *brahmacharya* helps us understand this original connotation. The root meaning of the Sanskrit word *Brahman* translates as "that which contains an inexhaustible potential of creativity." *Carya*, derived from the root *car*—"to walk," "to move," "to live"—means "the way of living." In *Glimpses of Raja Yoga*, Vimala Thakar explains that educating humans in perceiving, understanding, and becoming aware of the Divinity in all things was lost somewhere along the course of the English, German, or French translation, narrowing brahmacharya to the (still controversial and quite limiting) term "celibacy."[1] By recapturing the essence of brahmacharya as living a life dedicated to the awareness of Divinity, we naturally balance our imagined fears

---

1. Vimala Thakar, *Glimpses of Raja Yoga: An Introduction to Patanjali's Yoga Sutras* (Berkeley: Rodmell Press, 2005), 22-23.

of separateness and scarcity with the inexhaustible potential of the life source that surrounds us. We connect in meaningful ways to every aspect of life; we energetically expand and we open up to the boundless energy Patanjali promises with the practice of brahmacharya.

Patanjali gathered his knowledge from the teachings of ancient seers called *rishis*. These sages often lived in forests as interconnected members of their community. They taught "yoga" by example, living harmoniously with nature and members of their community. Nature was their teacher, and they, great students. Like Duke Senior in *As You Like It*, these sages found "tongues in trees, books in the running brooks, / Sermons in stones, and good in everything" (*As You Like It* 2.1). Their study was motivated by practical applications in everyday life, not just knowledge for knowledge's sake. They observed life closely (a skill often associated with great actors too), and their sensitivities grew. They brought forth universal truths with the intention of passing "yoga" on to future generations. Patanjali offers a series of sutras that serve as examples of what the ancient seers discovered by harmonizing with nature. Here are a few:

> Focusing with perfect discipline on the powers of an elephant or other entities, one acquires those powers.

> Focusing with perfect discipline on the sun yields insight about the universe.

> Focusing with perfect discipline on the moon yields insight about the stars' positions.

> (*Yoga Sutras* 3.25, 3.27, 3.28) [2]

---

2.   Hartranft, *Yoga-Sutra of Patanjali*, 53.

As a result of their respect for nature, rishis could see into realms of awareness inconceivable to us yet today—though steps toward evolving global consciousness are made daily!—and their heightened awareness of an all-pervasive Divine permeating everything shaped their existence.

Shakespeare's prolific use of nature provides an important backdrop for yoga lessons in appreciating the Divinity within and around us as inseparable sides of the same coin. As a place and an elemental force, nature is Shakespeare's great leveler. Nature is simultaneously mysterious and reliable in its ability to educate the moral imperatives that come with our place in the Great Chain of Being, a long-held belief in Shakespeare's day that held all matter and life to be an interconnected whole. This yoga-like theory about harmony and order in the universe positions humans uniquely between heaven and earth, God and a rock. In Shakespeare's plays and as yogis, we learn that our mission, should we choose to accept it, is to better orchestrate the glorious dance of our perceived duality of being mortal flesh and divine; to recognize the difference between the impermanence of illusion and the permanence of the spiritual interconnectedness of our inner and outer worlds.

Into the woods

Countless essays have been written on Shakespeare's use of nature: topics including nature as art, nature versus nurture, Shakespeare's horticulture, flower imagery in Shakespeare, and the like. Like the ancient seers, Shakespeare understood the profound ways nature mirrors our well-being. Many of his characters retreat to nature—a nearby woods, cave, hill, heath, or remote island will do—to alleviate the pressures of courtly life. For them, nature is employed as a place of refuge and redemption where lessons in mortality and morality are better integrated. Upon their return to society, or as they prepare to return, characters emerge clearly changed by any trials they have endured. The shift back and forth between the two worlds strikes an inner balance.

Take the main characters in *As You Like It*, for example. The heroine Rosalind, like Imogen in *Cymbeline* and Viola in *Twelfth Night*, dresses in the guise of a young man and renames herself (Ganymede) to escape her maniacal uncle (Duke Fredrick) and embraces the unknowns of living in the Forest of Arden.[3] Celia (Duke Fredrick's daughter) and the court jester Touchstone join her. For them, their flight into Arden is "in content / To liberty and not to banishment" (*As You Like It* 2.1). Other travelers, such as Orlando and Duke Senior, have also taken to the forest; the former for personal reasons, the latter as political safe haven. And let's not forget the pastoral folks who already live there. Despite their varying perceptions of the natural world and their motivations for being there, the Forest of Arden customizes lessons in love and life for all of them. Nature's trials promote self-growth and spiritual maturity while uniting its inhabitants as a communal whole. Marjorie Garber, author of *Shakespeare After All*, sums it up best:

> Many if not most of the characters in this play are overly concerned with self as they enter the Forest of Arden, and this mirroring forest and these mirroring debates give proportion and balance. Thus the forest socializes.[4]

The red center

In Shakespeare's plays, nature represents a journey inward, a willingness—or necessity, as the case may be—to courageously brave the unknowns of a transformational time and place. For us, one

---

3. Any association of Arden with Eden or Arcadia is purely intentional on Shakespeare's part; and, interestingly, it is also his mother's family birth name.
4. Marjorie Garber, *Shakespeare After All* (New York: Anchor Books, 2004), 447.

of two events tends to get us into nature's healing atmosphere: a relationship crisis (if even with our individual self), as is the case with many, if not most, Shakespearean characters; or a health crisis. Circumstances that enforce powering down the laptop and unplugging from the fear-induced dramas masquerading as news or self-identity help us to set aside our routine and honestly assess our habits. Yoga retreats in remote locations serve many. Millions find their local yoga studio an urban oasis or their backyard garden the ideal place to most naturally recalibrate. Others opt for a walking meditation: the rigors of the Pacific Crest Trail, a walkabout through the Australian desert, or a pilgrimage along Camino de Santiago (all of which have been made into films based on archetypal wanderers doing just that[5]).

Such was the case with me. Two years into the aftermath of a divorce and the disastrous attempts at dating again that followed, I took what felt a flying leap off a very tall cliff. I left a secure, stagnating career in corporate America and the frustrations of love to explore the Antipodes (Australia and New Zealand) for four months. The Red Center, as the heart of Australia is often called, became my Forest of Arden. Shedding baggage was my mission—a necessity really, as I arrived in Sydney on my fortieth birthday with three large suitcases, every imaginable pill to ward off dangerous tropical diseases, and a laptop computer neatly packed in my business briefcase. I could have been a cotraveler with Rosalind and her companions in a rendition of *As You Like It* that I saw at the Oregon Shakespeare Festival (2012), where they are first seen in the forest hauling a laughable amount of extraneous luggage. Touchstone lets his weighty load drop ceremoniously to the ground, (including Celia whom he's carrying on his back)—a hilarious, instructive moment that reflects our own unsubstantiated fears of lack in a world teeming with resources.

---

5. *Wild* (2014); *Tracks* (2013); *The Way* (2010).

But I digress. Four months on, carrying only a backpack (which my laptop fit into), I found myself staring out of a crowded, noisy caravan crossing the Outback on the Gunbarrel Highway. The term "highway" is a bit misleading, as it's an unpaved dirt road crisscrossed by wild camels. Cinnamon-red dust coated everything, including my hair and nostrils. After prior months of doing yoga on white sandy beaches, tramping the bush, and catching a fantastic performance of *A Midsummer Night's Dream* in Melbourne Royal Gardens, it was here, in an ordinary moment, staring out at the vast desert, exhausted from quasi-sleeping in a swag exposed to snakes, dingos, and spiders and digging ecologically sound long-drop toilets, that I finally heard my soul speak: "You're going to leave your job and move here." The details were a bit vague, but the heart of the message was spot-on.

Upon my return, I walked into my CEO's office, thanked him for a rewarding career with his company, and told him I was moving to New Zealand to open a yoga studio and write. That very same week (I kid you not) I met my future husband, who joined me in initiating three studios and nine teacher trainings Down Under. My modern-day-woman walkabout through Oz's natural wonderland had enabled me to hear—and trust—my true Self calling. Loud and clear.

Likewise, the characters of *As You Like It* are transformed in Arden, each according to an aspect of her or his reason for being there: Rosalind and Celia exchange controlling paternal figures for loving husbands; Orlando goes from tongue-tied, love-struck youth to articulate lover; Duke Senior regains his court; his brother, Duke Ferdinand, sees the errors of his ways; and comic and pastoral characters are matched and mated. Harmonious living—the true aim of yoga—is restored in Arden.

Dedicated time in nature teaches every step of the way. With conscious awareness, we find our way home to who we really are.

This requires dropping our baggage, literally and figuratively, if even a little bit at a time, and discovering that an inner strength empowers our lives. "There's no clock in the forest" (*As You Like It* 3.2), Orlando observes of Arden. When linear-thinking schedules are temporarily set aside and safety nets removed, our true thoughts and feelings find an opportunity to surface. Our minds are freed to roam. And, like Rosalind and Orlando, we can play, try on new roles, and discover new modes of self-expression. Nature's timelessness and its simple pleasures may take some getting used to, but they ultimately rebalance us. We remember that nature's cycles and rhythms are our cycles and rhythms; that all people have the same basic needs; and that even though our place in the Great Chain of Being, the Web of Life, is challenging, we somehow know that it is also a privileged experience designed to remind us of the necessity of listening to our souls. Shakespeare's plays remind us that a kind of off-the-mat yoga practice is always ready and waiting in nature's realm.

Don't mess with Mother Nature

In the BBC's *Shakespeare Retold* modern adaptation of *A Midsummer Night's Dream*, the ruffian fairy named Puck sums up his woodland world: "Nature is [pregnant pause] it's just so natural."[6] Meaning: Nature's elemental forces are powerful reflections of its inhabitants and unpredictable at best. Shakespeare employs nature as a mirroring force of mental-emotional conditions in many of his plays, most notably *The Tempest* and *King Lear*. In Puck's case, he refers to the effects of a contentious custody battle between his master, Oberon, and the fairy queen Titania. Their rocky marriage and serial infidelities are wreaking serious climatic change, as Titania herself readily admits:

---

6. *Shakespeare Retold, A Midsummer Night's Dream*, DVD, adapted by Peter Bowker, directed by Ed Fraiman (London: BBC, 2005).

Therefore the winds, piping to us in vain,
As in revenge, have suck'd up from the sea
Contagious fogs; which falling in the land
Have every pelting river made so proud
That they have overborne their continents.
(*A Midsummer Night's Dream* 2.1)

Twenty-two lines later, some of the most beautiful prose in the canon, she concludes that nature reflects their troubled behavior:

And this same progeny of evils comes
From our debate, from our dissension;
We are their parents and original. (2.1)

For the Vedic rishis, commercialization and profit were clearly not the aim of their relationship with the land. Respect for the Divinity in all things was paramount. As Shakespeare's yogis, Titania's passages remind us that how we treat our bodies and one another reflects how we treat the earth. The effects of pollution, climate change, and GMOs, although debated by some, indicate that a greater collective practice of brahmacharya is needed. We are, as the fairy queen notes, the "parents and original" responsible for our planet and the welfare of its inhabitants. Also like Oberon and Titania, we are fully capable of a midcourse correction. The practice of yoga is the magical change in consciousness that can help. Eliminating poverty, reducing unnecessary deforestation, xeriscaping, and simply consuming and recycling responsibly are efforts in the right direction.

Perfectly natural

Mortal or fairy, each of the main characters of *A Midsummer Night's Dream* is affected by and reflected in nature. And no one more so than Nick Bottom, a weaver turned amateur actor who, thanks to Puck, also has his head transformed into that of a braying ass. Bottom, however, also possesses the admirable ability to stay in the present moment with what happens in the Athenian woods. He is more than a body, a dramatically altered body at that. He is the only mortal character who is able to literally embrace nature's unpredictable changes. Instead of freaking out, he thrives. He is loved and loveable for being his authentic self.

As humans, we will eventually see our flesh sag, slow, and ultimately decay. Can we retain our equilibrium through these natural changes and remember that a spiritual power is always ready and waiting to embrace us just as we are? Or do we resist nature's beautiful patterns, including aging and alteration? By balancing the ego's compulsive abhorrence with dying (*abhinivesa*) with a dose of surrender and acceptance for our changing nature, we access the vitality life offers at any age. Respecting the Divinity in all things includes accepting the patterns of our natural body.

Likewise, when admiring an external view of natural beauty, we often spontaneously exclaim or text, "OMG!" Finding Divinity is easy when taking in the elegance of a warm, glowing sun rising over the African plains, or recalling the pranic om resonating in all things when we hear the humming of locust wings rising and falling with the ambient temperature. Brahmacharya is the choice to continually appreciate this same infinite, inexhaustible beauty in our messy internal landscapes and in the routine of our daily lives, as well.

Nature often brings out the natural foolishness of characters— think of Puck's amusement in *A Midsummer Night's Dream* when he laughs at "what fools these mortals be" (3.2). At the same time, a hard-won wisdom is often gained through a stripping down of the very fears and attachments that drive the characters there to begin with. Finding our equilibrium amidst the seeming chaos and confusion of life is an age-old balancing act that gets easier with the practice of brahmacharya. As with the Vedic rishis, nature is one of the Bard's favorite training grounds for teaching us that when everything falls apart, a newfound wisdom about who it is we really are lies not far behind. Sometimes this process can appear quite painful, as witnessed in *King Lear*, where nature strips attachments to false models of self-identity; other times, the experience is infused with laughter and ultimately ends with rejoicing, as in many of Shakespeare's comedies. The choice is, naturally, ours.

Aparigraha

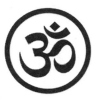

Nonpossessiveness

CHAPTER 13
Aparigraha as Reflected in *Macbeth*

We have all great cause to give great thanks.
–Coriolanus 5.4

Building on the spiritual practices of the previous four yamas—ahimsa, satya, asteya, and brahmacharya—is *aparigraha,*
or nonpossessiveness. This fifth and final yama necessitates
turning inward to develop a sense of gratitude and fulfillment for
everyday blessings: nutritious food, sanitary shelter, friendships,
health, and purposeful service. Beyond these basics, aparigraha
differentiates between what is truly needed and what is simply
an extraneous desire fueled by ego-motivated grasping. Choosing
wisely between needs that can be easily satisfied and desires that
only give rise to negative mental clutter is a conscious practice
requiring self-awareness and respect for the greater good.

And it's worth it. Patanjali promises a liberating sense of clarity
with the practice of aparigraha:

> Acknowledging abundance (Aparigraha), we recognize the
> blessings in everything and gain insights into the purpose for
> our worldly existence. (*Yoga Sutra* 2.39)[1]

Without aparigraha, however, what we do with our desires and
the ways our behavior affects others becomes a disorienting, futile
struggle in endless want. Our actions are fueled by thoughts
always demanding more—more love, more recognition, more
time, more material goods to adorn our bodies and homes, more

---

1. Devi, *Secret Power of Yoga*, 201.

money, et cetera. We suffer from an illusion of lack. Greed and a warped sense of entitlement can easily set in. Rather than enjoy the abundance we already have in the present moment, we are driven by a vicious cycle of exhausting behaviors and a distorted perception of future satisfaction.

Such is the case in Shakespeare's *Macbeth*, a play wholly about unchecked greed. A couple's ambitious rise to the top leaves a trail of bloody murders while simultaneously destroying their lives, illustrating the dangers of a complete disregard for aparigraha and its repercussions.

Altered states

The quick trajectory of the Macbeths' downward spiral emphasizes the slippery slope of destruction that comes with grasping and hoarding. Initially, Macbeth and Lady Macbeth merit political respect and well-earned offers of advancement and enjoy the strongest, most satisfying marriage in Shakespeare's entire canon. (Yes, I reckon even more so than Desdemona and Othello's or Romeo and Juliet's.) But due to a lack of gratitude for the fulfillment they have had, all is lost. Their greedy exploits breed crippling guilt, fear, and remorse.

With political ascent comes mental descent for the Macbeths. Sleeplessness and ugly hallucinations manifest. Conscious of his evil actions, though increasingly refusing to stop them, Macbeth finds himself unable to sleep restfully. In Act 2, Macbeth tells his wife he has murdered more than his predecessor (King Duncan) to gain his ill-won crown:

> Methought I heard a voice cry, "Sleep no more!
> Macbeth does murder sleep"—the innocent sleep,
> Sleep that knits up the raveled sleave of care. (*Macbeth* 2.2)

In Act 5, Lady Macbeth starts sleepwalking. As her self-regret for their gory affairs increases, her husband's need to protect his tenuous position grows bolder and bloodier. Throughout the play they are two sides of the same emotional teeter-totter. When Macbeth hesitates, his wife demands action. When Macbeth, a man once "full of the milk of human kindness," then turns monomaniacal in his quest to gain and retain power, his strong, articulate wife loses her mind. Increasingly estranged from each other, neither spouse perceives the other's terrible visions associated with their lethal avarice. Lady Macbeth can't see Banquo's ghost, though her husband certainly does; and Macbeth has no idea his wife is obsessed with washing a copious amount of King Duncan's imagined blood off her hands. What makes us shudder is how utterly avoidable these marital and mental breakdowns are, given the yogic practice of aparigraha. *Macbeth* makes us more discerning of how and why we obtain that which we seek, so that we are more able to avoid such unnecessary suffering.

As Shakespeare's yogis, we must begin where we are. Start on the mat: Do you watch others in yoga class and think to yourself, "I want that body. I want to be that teacher. I want this studio?" Taking care of the body and responsibly growing a yoga career are absolutely fine activities. But if such wishes and wants are rooted in covetousness, then discontentment fires up. Aparigraha weighs whether or not a desire warrants action, based on need. It questions the very nature of desire itself. Even a monk needs a bowl and a slat bed. But desires are, like ocean waves, limitless; one wave inexhaustibly gives rise to the next. When we appreciate the ability to do what we can with the body, tools, and time we've got, blessings in the present moment come rushing in. We feel free and peaceful.

Karma counts

Patanjali's *Yoga Sutra* 2.16 states:

Future suffering can and should be avoided.[2]

Macbeth and Banquo, a good army buddy of Macbeth (at first anyway), show how differently two people handle possessive thoughts.
Traveling back across moorland, victorious in a recent battle, they
encounter three witches who prophesize the future. A curious
Macbeth urges them to speak, to confirm his deepest, darkest
desire—that the crown shall encircle his head someday. And that
they do: the weird sisters predict Macbeth shall be named Thane of
Cawdor and then king; Banquo, although he shall not himself rule
in Scotland, will be father to future generations of kings.

It should be noted that Shakespeare's audiences believed in
witches. And although the noun "witches" can translate as "wise
women," most sixteenth- to seventeenth-century people considered them evil, especially royalty, who were terrified that their
supernatural powers could overturn a monarchy. Today's audiences tend to view the three witches as a modern-day equivalent of
astrologers who can read horoscopes, albeit spookier than most.
Then and now, patterns of destiny based on the alignment of the
stars at birth and "supernatural" powers (siddhis) are beliefs found
within yoga philosophy. The witches' ability to foresee events falls
squarely into this category of heightened sensitivities. Viewed
from a yogic perspective, the future, however, is ultimately up to
us. We plant the seeds that will grow with time.

As the play unfolds, Banquo and Macbeth both reflect on
the witches' predictions but act quite differently. Banquo is cast
as a foil to Macbeth; even if the prediction is true—which it
is—Banquo's "royalty of nature" is above foul play. Macbeth, on

---

2. Amey Mathews, "Future Suffering Can And Should be Avoided, Sutra 2.16,"
Yoga with Amey Mathews, Last modified 25 July 2006, http://www.yogawith-
amey.com/futuresuffering.html.

the other hand, morally misinterprets the witches' prophecies as legitimizing his fantasy of being king. He has always known that such advancement was loosely conceivable, although highly unlikely. But, by misconstruing fate, he unleashes an impatient lust for such power. His ego clinging supersedes his divine inner awareness. And we recognize the all-too-common humanness of such misguided belief.

When he is crowned King of Scotland, the spiritual implications of *parigraha*—unnecessary accumulating and hoarding, the opposite of aparigraha—naturally set in: Macbeth loses his peace of mind. With more power, he perceives only lack. He can't enjoy his reign because he's guilt-ridden about how he obtained it and he's too fearful about the possibility that it may be short-lived.

> Upon my head they placed a fruitless crown
> And put a barren scepter in my grip,
> Thence to be wrenched with an unlineal hand,
> No son of mine succeeding. (*Macbeth* 3.1)

The cumulative effect of Macbeth's greed is a sense of worthlessness. He literally struts and frets his last hour on the stage. Life to him becomes pretty bleak. "It is a tale / Told by an idiot, full of sound and fury, / Signifying nothing" (5.5). "The 'idiot' is the ego," and the guilt it lays on propels fruitless actions.[3] The Macbeths' violent acts simply have violent ends: Lady Macbeth commits suicide; and Macbeth has his head lopped off by Macduff, a man who, as the witches also later correctly predict, would not be of woman born. (As it turns out, he was from his mother's womb "untimely ripped" (5.3), a portent of Macbeth's imminent demise.)

---

3. Kenneth Wapnick, *Life, Death, and Love: Shakespeare's Great Tragedies and A Course in Miracles*, Vol 3: *Macbeth*, "*A Tale Told by an Idiot*" *The Murderous World of Guilt* (Temecula, Calif.: Foundation for A Course in Miracles, 2004), 1.

Banquo, on the other hand, doesn't survive the play, but the seeds of his noble thoughts and actions make him the father of a long line of kings. The purpose for his worldly existence lives on. Through the contrast between Macbeth and Banquo, we are advised that future suffering is avoidable, just as Patanjali counsels. Aparigraha reduces such future suffering, for ourselves and others. Otherwise, the blood and daggers of *Macbeth* become all too real.

We, like Shakespeare's characters, have choices—including the yama of aparigraha. How we behave possessing enhanced knowledge of our patterns and potentials sets our course for better or worse. An individual is not excused from acting morally simply because a few witches, a horoscope, or insider knowledge predicts dramatic change. Nor is such a prediction a green light to awaken the dark side of the self to criminally force the prediction to happen without dire consequence.

With every choice, the body and soul accumulate particles of karma, a less-remembered consequence of possessiveness. This yogic principle of causality is played out onstage and beyond in *Macbeth*. This play warns us that prospering by the deception of others ultimately weakens the moral fiber of those perpetrating such acts, often with negative ramifications that can span generations. Macbeth's tragic flaw is that he is well aware of the choices before him, and yet he commits murder in the name of ambition despite a guilty conscience.

Conscious of Shakespeare's yogic lesson, we can choose aparigraha as the antidote to unregulated possessiveness. At any point, we can pause in our pursuit of more _____ (fill in the blank). We can replace what we want with an appreciation for what we have. And whenever gratitude (the corresponding niyama of santosha, or contentment) replaces scarcity mentality, we are happier. The repercussions of guilt are exchanged with the glories of a purposeful existence. It doesn't take three witches to tell us that.

CHAPTER 14
Aparigraha as Reflected in *Timon of Athens*

Superfluity [having too much] *comes sooner by white hairs,*
but competency [having just enough] *lives longer.*
—*The Merchant of Venice* 1.2

In the summer of 2015, I caught New Zealand's first performance of *Timon of Athens* in 150 years. I repeat: 150 years! And some festivals "round out" their performances of the entire canon by including *Timon* in the lineup only then. Arguably, *Timon* has never been one of Shakespeare's most widely known, beloved, or frequently performed plays, even in his lifetime. There's no romantic subplot in *Timon*, and the humor is certainly there, but it's dark and deeply satirical. And, as Shakespeare doesn't sugarcoat anything, he obviously wasn't about to begin to do so in a play all about money mongers. That said, there is absolutely every reason to fully embrace this play, especially from a yogic perspective. Timon's drama and the direction it takes provide a precious reminder of the importance of aparigrapha (nonpossessiveness) in every socio-economic era. It is a well-written, fascinating snapshot of the human condition when it comes to money, politics, and power—a lesson in Shakespeare's yoga needed now perhaps more than ever.

I want you to want me
Timon, an Athenian noble, struggles with money management and what it means. He wastes a fortune on extravagant gifts and lavish parties for a large circle of self-serving admirers, mostly artists,

politicians, and merchants seeking patronage. And if someone gives him a gift, it's widely known that "he repays / Sevenfold above itself" (*Timon of Athens* 1.1). This isn't philanthropy; it's craziness. Financial suicide. A "churlish philosopher" named Apemantus tries to warn him:

> Thou givest so long,
> Timon, I fear me thou wilt give away thyself in
> paper shortly: what need these feasts, pomps and
> vain-glories? (1.2)

Timon's deeply entrenched habit of buying admiration blinds him to Apemantus's bitter truths. And, sure enough, Timon's faithful accountant, Flavius, soon informs him that he's flat-out broke, and his "friends" quickly abandon him. One by one, they rebuke his request for financial aid with excuses so flimsy that even Timon's messengers are appalled by their hypocrisy. For example: Flaminus, one of Timon's servants, arrives at the home of one of Timon's so-called friends, Lucullus, carrying a box that Timon readily assumes will return filled with a cash loan. Initially Lucullus assumes the box contains a gift from Timon. (Oh the irony!). When instead Flaminus requests the loan on Timon's behalf, not only is the loan denied, but Lucullus tries to bribe the servant with a wink and some coins to say they never spoke. Disgusted, Flaminus departs, but not before hurling the coins back at Lucullus. Two more such episodes follow. The chips are down and Timon's former admirers suddenly want absolutely nothing to do with him.

This play being thematically similar to *King Lear*, the play Shakespeare was to write next, Timon chooses self-banishment in response to gross ingratitude. In stark contrast to Lear's epiphanies, however, Timon spends his remaining days as a misanthropic recluse, engaging in a destructive form of self-definition in which he justifies his resolute hatred for all mankind.

> Timon will to the woods, where he shall find
> Th' unkindest beast more kinder than mankind . . . .
> And grant, as Timon grows, his hate may grow
> To the whole race of mankind, high and low,
> Amen. (4.1)

That may sound drastic, but it happens.

What's unusual is that, while digging for roots to eat near his cave, Timon discovers a trove of gold. (What are the chances, right? But that too happens, in Shakespeare, anyway.) Only now, Timon considers gold the "yellow slave" that undoes religions and curses the blessed. No good can come of it, in his mind. Nonetheless, word of his reversal of fortune spreads quickly (no surprise there). His solitary world is suddenly punctuated with a steady stream of returning "friends" and visitors, all of whom, whether they deserve it or not, Timon now rebukes with disdain. His vilification of "ingrateful man" (4.3) becomes an unshakeable vow of contempt that eventually entombs his body and soul.

Shakespeare's audiences would not have been at all surprised by the hero's tragic outlook on life, because for the longest time the name Timon had cultural associations with the term "misanthrope." Hence, even before they entered the theater, the title was a dead-give away that Timon's transformation was going to end badly for him. The question was: How would it happen? Watching his fate unfold would be the real draw. Over 400 years later, this is still a play that certainly leaves you thinking: *How can I best react to life's disappointments? Does my perception of others and of life itself reflect how I see myself? How do flattery and greed fan the flames of want on a socio-economic level? Where in my yogic lifestyle can I make better choices than Timon by practicing aparigraha?*

Possessed

When it comes to accumulating possessions, most people think of material goods, wealth, relationships, or power. Timon's story teaches us that perceiving such possessions as an extension of self-worth fosters a dangerous illusion. Waste and overspending are cautionary indicators that such trouble is brewing, as highlighted in the play's opening acts. According to yoga philosophy, a less-considered form of possession is wallowing in low thoughts or negative emotions—anger, fear, hate, jealousy, and the like—exactly the type of negative mental clutter that eventually derails Timon.

The word "want" appears thirteen times in *Timon*, significantly more than in any other Shakespearean play. Whether he's playing the role of philanthropist or misanthrope, Timon sabotages himself by enabling his extreme wants to pen in his psyche. Timon's first spoken line foreshadows this tragic flaw. With trumpeted fanfare, thronged by admiring hangers-on, he enters the party commenting, "Imprisoned is he, say you?" (1.1). From beginning to end, Timon is the real prisoner, a prisoner of conscience. Mentally and emotionally, he's trapped by his perceived possessions, whether it's meaningless gifts, false friends, or pessimistic thoughts. The problem is, he doesn't realize that aparigraha is the key to his release.

Instead, he cynically philosophizes on the nature of want with anyone who dares approach his cave, including thieves looking to lighten his load of gold.

TIMON

Why should you want? Behold, the earth hath roots;
Within this mile break forth a hundred springs;
The oaks bear mast, the briers scarlet hips;
The bounteous housewife, nature, on each bush
Lays her full mess before you. Want! why want?

FIRST THIEF

We cannot live on grass, on berries, water,

As beasts, and birds, and fishes.

TIMON

Nor on the beasts themselves, the birds, and fishes;

You must eat men. (4.3)

It's a real dog-eat-dog world according to Timon now. Spotlighting the hero's pessimistic worldview, some modern directors collaborate with designers to create mobster-period or animal-themed costuming. The production I watched in New Zealand employed the latter; the student actors of Victoria University of Wellington wore animal masks in several scenes. In 2008, director Lucy Bailey and designer William Dudley draped netting over the stage of Shakespeare's Globe, through which actors, vulture-like, swooped like parasites on Timon. Point made: mankind can be barbaric.

But does such direction serve? Is Timon simply reduced to a victim of his external circumstances? Does this interpretation sidetrack the fact that his wasteful spending and inner longing for flattery got him into this state? Do we agree with Timon's (and Apemantus's) ongoing metaphors that unilaterally reduce humans to "affable wolves, meek bears" (3.6)?

The true beauty of Shakespeare's plays is that we leave the theater thinking the world will be different. Better somehow. Even after a dark play such as *Timon*. This is where yoga comes in. When watching *Timon* through the lens of aparigraha, we rest assured his choices created his karma, not the other way around. We are vividly reminded that, like Timon, our life is merely a stage on which we're acting out our deeds (karma). The story of our lives is just a play unfolding. It's a performance we are each personally directing and starring in at the same time. Practicing non-possessiveness (and the other four yamas) shifts the performance spotlight from the ego to the higher Self, something Timon fails to do—spectacularly. Aparigraha encourages us to let go of who we think we are as bodies, as bank accounts, as reputations. And as yogis, we experience a reality check when even the trappings of spiritual materialism that honor only "my brand of yoga" come up.

Greed negatively impacts us all. In that respect, Timon was absolutely right. But, through the practice of aparigraha, rather than run and hide like Timon, we wake up to what's happening in the world and do what we can as Shakespeare's yogis to make a positive difference.

Enough already

Timon translates all too easily to the economic injustice parading as permissible capitalism today. Income inequality in America is at an all-time high. A sane, healthy life-work balance grows harder to maintain. And many families live paycheck-to-paycheck, relying on credit and second and third jobs to make ends meet. The stupefying disparity between the uberwealthy one percent and the rest of society cautions disaster for democracy. Movies like *The Big Short* (2015), *The Wolf of Wall Street* (2013) and documentary films such as *Inequality for All* (2013) and *Inside Job* (2010) expose an indefensible reality that should shake us awake. In addition, statistics show that many Americans are stuffing their homes to the point that a 24 billion–dollar self-storage industry has emerged to house extra belongings. As a society, are we like Timon, enabling corporate greed and hoarding as a way of life? Are possessions possessing us?

Yoga is now a mega-multibillion-dollar industry with over 20 million practitioners in the United States alone. If the growing trend is to do the greatest good both physically and spiritually, it behooves us to consider the economic impact of yoga consumerism—mats, water bottles, specialty towels, designer clothing, and hundred-dollar-a-day juice fasts, for example. Are the products we procure manufactured by globally responsible sources? Do we respect the store's social and environmental impact? Do we really need the product? And, if so, can we donate or recycle the used item it replaces? How does our practice reflect the joy of less? These simple applications of aparigraha are yoga, a spiritual practice that takes time and discernment.

Aparigraha is the willingness to face the inconvenient truths about our everyday apportionments of what is enough. It's about opening our cupboards and closets recognizing the overflowing abundance we have. It's gaining a growing awareness of the ego's desiring clamor and simply responding, "Enough already." Perhaps most important, it's an eagerness to responsibly share with those who are less fortunate. Our highest achievement becomes making sure fair trade, opportunity, and equable standards apply universally and are upheld. What we want more than anything else is that our families, businesses, nation, and world are vibrant and healthy for everyone, and we're willing to participate in their creation one conscious action at a time for as many lifetimes as it takes. In the process, aparigraha makes our souls feel lighter, almost immediately. A freedom arises from within and without.

Despite the many myths about yoga, it's most often *not* about living in a cave, eating meager vegetation, clothed in a loincloth and spouting philosophy like Timon; it's a dedication to the choices that unify us as essentially loving beings.

Imagine

Leave it to the Bard to represent all angles of any human condition. If Timon paints a picture of mankind at its worst, then Gonzalo in *The Tempest* counterpoints with a vision of a living utopia—a time and place where everyone is provided for. Want is no longer an issue. Aparigraha is a way of life.

I' th' commonwealth I would by contraries
Execute all things; for no kind of traffic
Would I admit; no name of magistrate;
Letters should not be known; riches, poverty,
And use of service, none; contract, succession,
Bourn, bound of land, tilth, vineyard, none;
No use of metal, corn, or wine, or oil;
No occupation; all men idle, all;
And women too, but innocent and pure;
No sovereignty;
[...]
All things in common nature should produce
Without sweat or endeavour: treason, felony,
Sword, pike, knife, gun, or need of any engine,
Would I not have; but nature should bring forth,
Of its own kind, all foison, all abundance,
To feed my innocent people. (*The Tempest* 2.1)

Gonzalo is rudely mocked for his optimism by the other characters onstage, power-hungry politicos who masterminded usurping the Duke of Milan (now, Prospero) twelve years ago. These are men who epitomize Timon's animalistic worldview.

Gonzalo's virtues are not lost on those who appreciate his visionary ideas, however. In the act prior, Prospero praised this kind, old man for his generous deeds and foresight when Prospero and his baby daughter were exiled. And today, one cannot help but wonder if yogi John Lennon directly echoes Gonzalo's words in these popular lyrics to his song "Imagine":

Imagine there's no countries
It isn't hard to do
Nothing to kill or die for
And no religion too

Imagine all the people
Living life in peace...
You may say I'm a dreamer
But I'm not the only one
I hope someday you'll join us
And the world will be as one
Imagine no possessions
I wonder if you can
No need for greed or hunger
A brotherhood of man
Imagine all the people
Sharing all the world.[1]

Like the Beatles song, Gonzalo's utopia speech raises the bar for humanity. It asks us to drop our carefully guarded boundaries and live as the interdependent beings we are; to trust that nature, including human nature, knows how to provide for its own, and that every single creature is innately worthy of sharing in life's bounty. Knowing that this peaceful vision is still clouded by war, poverty, and oppression, where do those of us who believe in the power of our united goodness find footing? How do we balance Timon's commentary on greed with Gonzalo's faith in a shared abundance?

Thirteenth-century Sufi poet Rumi wisely suggests, "Out beyond our ideas of right-doing and wrong-doing, there is a field. I'll meet you there."[2]

Both the theater and the yoga studio make ideal fields.

Sacred spaces

I wouldn't consider myself especially sentimental. Nonetheless, as I cozied into my lawn chair parked in the Boston Common,

---

1. John Lenon, *Imagine*, Song (Ascot: Ascot Sound Studios, 1971).
2. Coleman Barks, trans., *The Essential Rumi* (San Francisco: HarperOne, 2004).

observing thousands of people gather one evening in 2013 to watch *The Two Gentlemen of Verona*, tears pooled up. How is it that attending a Shakespeare play has this effect on me? (*Again*, I might add. Okay, maybe I'm more sentimental than I let on.) I asked myself: *Could it be that, three months after a lethal bomb ripped through the psyche of the city during its famous marathon, here we all were, happily unloading our backpacks for a preshow picnic on the grass (with no visible security, body searches, or devices to scan for weapons of mass destruction)? Was it because of our united purpose: to laugh and learn how we behave as friends (a major theme of* Two Gents*)? Or was it because Shakespeare clearly understood the powerful impact of peacefully trying to make sense of our similarities through play instead of tearing one another apart over our differences with war? Perhaps my tears were proof of the inherent happiness we feel when, to paraphrase Noble Peace Prize winner Thich Nhat Hanh, we awaken from our illusion of separateness.* In any case, the play's the thing that harmoniously brought thousands together that summer evening. And with the closing line, "One feast, one house, one mutual happiness" (*The Two Gentlemen of Verona* 5.4), the actors and audience gave each other a standing ovation—through which I dripped a few more happy sentimental tears and the stars twinkled.

Shakespeare's teaching vehicle of the theater is well chosen. A cultural community is born of uniting people for a higher purpose: actors with audiences, dramaturges with technicians and designers, dancers with musicians, ticket sellers with marketers, twenty-first-century directors with Elizabethan playwrights, et cetera. In yoga as with theater, interconnecting with other complex human beings ignites the power of *satsang* (spending time with like-minded individuals or groups who share the same truth). In the interdependent experience we find support and reassurance.

We are also more likely confronted with situations that will test and temper the truth, a healthy uncomfortableness that we may not as readily encounter in rehearsing solo acts or in a solitary yoga practice (as wonderful and important as those two experiences are). Interruptions temper our need for uniformity when sharing a practice space with others. Coughs, farts, verbal outbursts . . . I've heard them all in yoga class, at the theater, and onstage. (Sir Toby Belch in *Twelfth Night* can produce all such sounds generously. Playing his cohort and love interest, Maria, in the Texas summer heat prepared me very well for hot yoga.) Tears, sweat, and laughter are also just as likely in yoga class as they are at any theater production. A good field is oftentimes a messy place.

Shawn Sides, award-winning director of The Rude Mechanicals, an Austin-based theater company, comments on the importance of believing in the interdependent nature of the creative process despite inevitable disappointments and disagreements. She observes, "We can't make anything good until we make a hundred terrible things and that takes a lot of time; time that, in the moment, feels 'wasted.' And we can't make one hundred failures until we get the whole posse in the room, failing together."[3] Likewise, there is no such thing as a perfect yoga class. (That's why it's called a practice.)

Every day, more and more students come to the mat for wide and varied reasons, all of them equally valid. Through skillful instruction and class commitment these sessions bring practitioners into a perceptible whole. Sometimes the room sounds like one big, breathing lung. It's a little slice of what we're capable of on a grander scale.

This same experience intensifies in the yoga teacher training process. As a trainer for many years I regularly witnessed somewhat nervous individuals arrive for the first day of training. Many often thought they had little in common with the other

---

3. *Doris Duke Performing Artist Awards*, "Shawn Sides," 2015, http://ddpaa.org/artist/shawn-sides/

twenty-three trainees seated around them, or so they told me later. (Fast-forward five months of training.) The collective commitment—to learn more about yoga, themselves, and how to pass along their truth to others—never failed in transforming these same individuals, even the skeptical ones, into a cohesive family of friends. And into confident yoga teachers, as well, each unique. Every training season reminded me, so much, of what I loved most as a performer at Shakespeare at Winedale: the contagious solidarity that courses through the blood when the spirit of play makes all the hard work, the many trials and momentary tears, into something no one individual could have ever created or experienced without the others. It's the feeling of something very, very present. A mutual joy. A shared courage. The bar on the potential of collective creativity stays permanently raised for the rest of your life.

When working with his actors, Shakespeare himself would have felt this same collective selfhood, the experience of blending identities—every player having his own part but depending upon the others to succeed as a cohesive whole. In yoga philosophy any process that activates our unity of being can be called *advaita*. The playwright clearly appreciated the play as such a self-realization device. It requires that ego trips take a backseat to the troupe's collective purpose, and in doing so stimulates advaita, the realization of the oneness of who we are. Many of his plays incorporate a play within the play (most notably *A Midsummer Night's Dream* and *Hamlet*). Thematically, Shakespeare also shows how putting on a play and the act of playing itself emphasize an inherently nondualistic experience. Meaning, what happens onstage is simply a reflection of the characters' own story—and ours, too, as actors on the stage of life, united by the ties that make our differences unimportant and indistinguishable.

During their initial training session, I aimed to pass that synergistic baton on to the yoga teacher trainees, adding this guidance, "Becoming a yoga teacher is ultimately about being a more present person, with your Self and others." That, followed by the advice our summer theater Shakespeare professor (Dr. James Ayres, "Doc" we call him) so often gave us, a line from *The Winter's Tale*: "It is required you do awake your faith" (5.3).

Over time, when theaters and yoga studios are seasoned with the energy of aparigraha—a willingness to share resources, time, space, ideas, dialogue, breakdowns, and breakthroughs —purposeful words and actions arise. As a result, a yoga studio morphs into a theater of transformation, and a theater becomes a communal training ground on the power of yogic principles. Inspired by the exploration into our shared humanity, they become fields filled with the faith of our highest potential. They grow in power. They invoke a palpable reverence the moment we enter them. And, ultimately, no one leaves these sacred spaces the same as they were when they entered.

Imagine that.

CHAPTER 15
Aparigraha as Reflected in
The Merchant of Venice

How far that little candle throws its beams!
So shines a good deed in a naughty world.
—The Merchant of Venice 5.1

At the start of a yoga practice, setting an intention is recommended and regularly prompted by teachers. Palms softly unite just in front of the heart (a symbolic hand gesture called *anjali mudra*) or hands rest in an alternative meditative position. As minds center on the purpose at hand, practice is dedicated to an individual or group in need of support. Many studios hold special yoga classes specifically to raise money or awareness for the betterment of society: finding cures for diseases, aiding disaster relief efforts, or alleviating suffering in some meaningful way. Events such as *yoga malas* (108 poses, chants, or prayers) are also organized to raise the collective consciousness and free our world of suffering. Dedicating the fruits of our yogic practice to improve others' lives, not just our own, transforms them into offerings, prayers in motion. It activates trust in a Universal Power (God, Buddha, Mother Nature, Brahman, etc.), making us instruments of peace. It's aparigraha (nonpossessiveness) at its best. And, as with all yamas, when our choices ease others' pain, they naturally instill a more loving and harmonious relationship with our self. It's a spiritual win-win.

Without aparigraha, however, we can become stubbornly attached to an attitude of "What's in it for me?" even during a series of Sun Salutations. In such moments, we may tone our body but lose the inherent benefits of yoga's divinely inspired higher purpose. Our postures become an exercise in collecting rewards rather than a process of self-liberation. Not to mention, we are also more likely to push ahead when we or our students are injured, sick, or tired, increasing the likelihood of injury.

The repercussions of grasping at things even if they are "rightfully" ours are also the focus of Shakespeare's *The Merchant of Venice*. In the play's fourth act, lessons in the importance of aparigraha reach a dramatic climax.

Mercy me

Envision a courtroom setting. Shylock, a Jewish moneylender, is entitled by law to claim repayment from Antonio, the titular merchant of Venice. Their contract clearly states that if the bond is not repaid by Antonio on time, as the case now stands, Shylock can demand his due: a pound of flesh. Human flesh. And it is "to be by him [Shylock] cut off / Nearest the merchant's heart" (*The Merchant of Venice* 4.1). Enter Portia (the heroine disguised as a young male lawyer). Given the rather strange and lethal terms of the bond, Portia advises the Jew to be merciful, to surrender his suit for the sake of a higher cause:

> The quality of mercy is not strain'd,
> It droppeth as the gentle rain from heaven
> Upon the place beneath: it is twice blest;
> It blesseth him that gives and him that takes.
> [...]
> Though justice be thy plea, consider this—
> That in the course of justice none of us
> Should see salvation. We do pray for mercy,
> And that same prayer doth teach us all to render
> The deeds of mercy. (4.1)

"Mercy" is not a word we use that much anymore. Instead, we use words like "forgiveness" and "compassion." Whatever term you prefer, Portia's speech is yogic counsel on the merits of practicing aparigraha—letting go of the mental-emotional impulse to win at any cost, to prove our point, or to get even, as Shylock's underlying motive appears to be. Retribution, anger, and pride underscore Shylock's responses in court and the terms of the bond itself. But why?

As witnesses to these proceedings, we bear in mind that throughout his life Shylock has been maligned by prejudice and oppression—the hoarding of negative opinion or control over others. He has been spat upon and called dog for being Jewish and for his occupation of usury, including, admittedly, by Antonio.

Shylock is not the only social outcast, though. Complex issues surrounding homosexuality, female subjugation, racial stereotyping, and the high stakes of living on credit mutate all around Venice and Belmont (Portia's hometown), cause havoc and heartache throughout the play. Social and spiritual imbalances permeate the interior landscape of most every character. Therefore, Portia's advice on the healing power of mercy is a poignant lesson, not just for Shylock, but for everyone in court. And that includes us.

Like Shylock, we have deeply ingrained emotional ties, often culturally trained, to the impulse to take our pound of flesh. To be the most correct. To be the most successful. To be however the culture most wants us to see ourselves, regardless whether it's at the expense of others or our own self-negation. Even in yoga circles, these misperceptions are the ego's definition of power living, and they backfire pain and suffering.

But when new habits like mercy start to flow freely in our lives, when they're "not strain'd" (meaning not forced) and practically habitual, it's blessings all around. Yoga is now working through us. Our lives become a source of connection rather than separation.

Portia reminds us mercy flows as freely as rain if we let it. With aparigraha, perspectives in thought and behavior gradually shift. When we start choosing forgiveness rather than holding a grudge, our relationships evolve. When we let go of the need to be right all the time, we naturally convey more openness. By gracefully being who we are rather than who others define us as, greater freedom is created for everyone. When we chip away at the deadly bonds of prejudice, we bask in the abundance of a universal oneness. Clearing our hearts and minds of violent thoughts and feelings is aparigraha, powerful yoga.

The case continues

Portia's reminder on the healing power of mercy echoes Patanjali's guidance on the courageous, conscious practice of Pratipaksha Bhavana.

> When presented with disquieting thoughts or feelings, cultivate an opposite, elevated attitude. This is Pratipaksha Bhavana. (*Yoga Sutra* 2.33)[1]

Pratipaksha Bhavana is yoga for the mind. And it works. We encounter this same yogic practice in *The Tempest* when Prospero consciously reverses his acts of vengeance with the virtue of forgiveness. Not so with Shylock, though. As Act 4 of *Merchant* plays out, Shylock's tragic flaw arises out of his inability to shake off his fixation on collecting a pound of Antonio's flesh. His troubled heart and mind never cultivate a gentler answer.

Despite Portia's initial plea for mercy, Shylock refuses to budge: "There is no power in the tongue of man / To alter me. I stay here on my bond" (*The Merchant of Venice* 4.1). Shylock wants what's his, exactly as the contract provides; and he's brought a knife and

---

1. Devi, *Secret Power of Yoga*, 171.

scales (but, glaringly, no surgeon) in his determination to get it. He even refuses financially advantageous and legally acceptable alternatives to his lethal restitution, including an offer of three times the sum Antonio originally owed him. Shylock craves only the law, the penalty, and the fulfillment of this (very bizarre, but entirely legitimate) contract. Cultivating an opposite attitude appears beyond his grasp.

Until the tables turn on him. As Shylock prepares to cut Antonio's exposed chest, Portia adds one last legal reminder:

> There is something else.
> This bond doth give thee here no jot of blood.
> The words expressly are "a pound of flesh."
> Take then thy bond, take thou thy pound of flesh,
> But in the cutting it if thou dost shed
> One drop of Christian blood, thy lands and goods
> Are by the laws of Venice confiscate
> Unto the state of Venice (4.1)

Of course, cutting flesh without drawing a drop of blood is impossible. It's probably literature's most famous legal loophole, and one that saves Antonio's life while sealing Shylock's fate.

The Jew now finds *himself* at the mercy of others, namely the Christian court and Antonio. The Venetian judge tempers justice with mercy, but not by much. The very mercy asked of Shylock just moments ago is now, ironically, mostly denied to him. By the end of the proceedings Shylock is stripped of everything he holds most dear: his ducats, his daughter, and his religious community. In addition to court fines, half of Shylock's estate is awarded to Antonio, who, in turn, offers to give it back to Shylock but only if he converts to Christianity and bequeaths all his goods to his daughter, Jessica (who has long since secretly eloped with Lorenzo, a Christian). The Jew's severe forfeitures make for a problematic comedy, an uneasy "happy" ending—and rightly so. Double standards are blatant. A vicious cycle of prejudice and oppression perpetuates itself. Could the legal system have considered a more equitable and evolved resolution?

Likewise, what if Shylock had practiced aparigraha instead of insisting on "justifiable" restitution? What if he had cultivated an attitude opposite that of uncompromising hard-heartedness? From a yogic perspective, his choice of more enlightened actions would have been (as Portia describes earlier) "an attribute to God himself" (4.1), blessing both himself and others. Shylock would have also departed the courtroom exceedingly better off than when he entered—materially and spiritually. The abundance Patanjali promises with the fifth and final yama, nonpossessiveness, would have naturally manifested. Instead, Shylock exits, uttering, "I am not well" (4.1), promising to sign the court settlement.

If after *Merchant* we leave the theater a bit uneasy, Shakespeare has done his job as a yoga teacher. The play's psychologically complex characters and challenging themes make us, as in any good yoga class, comfortably uncomfortable, prompting us to turn inward and reexamine our lives. We grow in awareness that when any one of us suffers under the stress of power imbalances or a corrupted interdependence, we are all affected; and that mindlessly taking "what's mine" without regard for the welfare of others is one of the unkindest cuts of all.

Character development

One of the amazing things about Shakespeare is the way characters like Shylock continue to reflect both the times and how we view ourselves as spiritually evolved beings sharing a common human experience. Post-World War II audiences sensitive to the atrocities of Nazi anti-Semitism may be surprised to learn that it wasn't until the nineteenth century that actors first began to portray Shylock as the abused, semi-tragic figure he is today. Until then, he was cast and costumed as a comic character or the Devil incarnate, as was likely the case in Shakespeare's own time. In the 1930s, anti-Semitics used the play to further justify their hatred of Jews. As with yoga, however, exploring our human condition means taking in the many aspects of our self, "warts and all." Shakespeare was very comfortable and adept at that. What we do with our disquieted thoughts and feelings is the crux of spiritual evolution—and of the timeless adaptability of his literary masterpieces. Historical interpretations of Shylock and the long list of Shakespeare's other multidimensional characters indicate our progress on the path to enlightenment.

Some of Shakespeare's characters are loosely based on historical figures or derived from former literary works. Shylock, for example, was most likely the Bard's literary twist on a theatrical villain named Barabas and the title role of *The Jew of Malta*, a popular play in Shakespeare's day by Christopher Marlowe. Although Shakespeare's rendition of his characters makes them not "real" at all, their stories are so like our own that we often refer to and think of them as such. Othello, Rosalind, Romeo, Cordelia, Falstaff, Beatrice and Benedict, Hal, Hamlet, and many others (most on a first name basis) are intrepid explorers who've "been there"—to the very center of life's most varied and complex human dilemmas, repeatedly. And because their adventures in being human, like the yamas, transcend time, place, gender, and race, we continue to project ourselves into their words and actions. Eventually, we will learn those same universal lessons and no longer need to stage them. Our remembrance will be complete and we will reside once again in the good ol' days of the Golden Age of Enlightenment (*Satya Yuga*).

As that golden age is still before us, according to human perceptions of time, anyway, we bear in mind that "all the world's a stage" (*As You Like It* 2.7) for our yoga practice; that when we act in opposition to the principles of ethical living, the quality of life is negatively impacted; and that when we consciously live in tribute to our highest being, we promote harmony in the world and in our self. Along the way, we begin to include, rather than distance ourselves from, the contradictory nature of life. We find peace in acknowledging and accepting both the human and spiritual sides of our selves more clearly, more wholly, and more compassionately.

Shakespeare reminds us that our roles are forever unfolding and interchangeable, and that "one man in his time plays many parts" (2.7). We are potentially *every* part of *every* character we see or play, onstage and on the yoga mat. In yoga class, each posture (asana) represents a changeable dimension of our physicality—a reflection of our inner resolve or turmoil, or the potential for peace between the two, on any given day. Like Shakespeare's characters, we also have the power to interpret our role differently at any given moment. So, when the seasons of our practice shift, when we can no longer access a difficult headstand, or perhaps attain it for the first time, we are okay either way. We develop *true* character and become increasingly comfortable with our leading role as Shakespeare's yogis: that of rainmakers, cultivators of mercy, forgiveness, and compassion in our relationships with our self and one another.

Because there's nothing more blessed than a gentle rain when and where it's needed most.

Conclusion

I would we were all of one mind, and one mind good.
—*Cymbeline* 5.4

Yoga philosophy and Shakespeare may initially strike us as serious stuff, but by heeding their spiritual wisdom we enjoy a happier life. We are more aware of the illusionary thoughts that lead us to believe that we are anything but whole and interconnected.

Despite massive amounts of conflicting, often negative information about our bodies and our world, and the fears and anxieties we may create in our mind as a result, we know on a gut level there is an inherent goodness and unified mind, or consciousness, we all share. We are simply learning to believe and trust in that abundant wholeness once again. Yoga practice opens these channels of remembrance. Spending time with Shakespeare does, too. His version of our experience on this great globe is timeless and amazingly timely. He presents a provocative and well-rounded picture of what's really happening—internally and externally, universally and metaphysically, then and now. His yogic viewpoints improve our outlook on life: he shows us that the laws of cause and effect are to be heeded; the inherent contradictions found within every major character's words and actions paint a fuller, richer picture of who we are; he raises questions that make us think twice before answering; and he portrays looking foolish as living authentically rather than as personal failure or an embarrassing mistake.

Play after play, Shakespeare inspires our faith in the ways of right living. His works present universal truths that directly correspond to Patanjali's ancient guidance of the five yamas—ahimsa (nonviolence), satya (truthfulness), asteya (nonstealing), brahmacharya (balance and moderation), and aparigraha (nonpossessiveness). Shakespearean theater and yoga philosophy prove complementary sources of spiritual wisdom designed to awaken us from the dream of separation from the Self. They also remind us how precious our collective consciousness is, how powerful it can be, and how good it feels to be of "one mind, and of one mind good" (*Cymbeline* 5.4). And sometimes we laugh, sometimes we cry, as both are the outpourings of our heart when the poignant remembrance of who we are and how we feel when we are whole again is in play.

Let's get metaphysical

The stars shine big and bright in the Texas countryside. Though most of the audience had departed, I could still hear the laughter of those reluctant to leave the theater barn, most likely former students of the summer Shakespeare program I was now in. Alone on an old, handcrafted bench behind the theater, I felt an evaporation of the various characters I had played that weekend: Mistress Page, Gratiano, and Second Merchant (of Ephesus), amongst other smaller roles. This mélange of Shakespearean characters was lifting off my being and fading into that vast night sky. It felt like a peeling of personas, cleansing and peaceful. Only latent impressions remained and do so until this day.

I have never forgotten that unique sensation nor the deep contentment for having lived so many colorful lives in such a short amount of time that summer so long ago. If I had experienced formal meditation or a savasana (Corpse Pose) by that age— which wasn't to happen for another ten years yet—I would have said that expansive inner glow felt a lot like yoga. I sensed there was a part of me that was genderless, ageless, and as infinitely connected to all things of all time as the bright stars high above. I couldn't articulate it yet, but I inwardly acknowledged that there was something transcendent about existence: that any role we play in life is merely a temporary experience or, as the Bard describes, "such stuff / As dreams are made on" (*The Tempest* 4.1); and that surrendering to, rather than resisting, the inevitability of our temporal state makes us happier. Today that means that even the pageantry of yoga studios, gurus, students, books, and water bottles will—poof—dissolve. And that's okay. Letting go of our attachments is one of the very reasons we practice yoga to begin with.

Playing Shakespeare as a youth (followed by passion for attending Shakespearean theater) prepared me in so many ways for the yoga experience and for sharing it with others. It taught me humility, about the repetitive nature of humor, and how to listen with my whole body. I can recognize the difference between acting and playing—the former smacks of artificiality; the latter connects words from one's soul to another's. A room full of yoga students harmonizing with an opening om still feels a lot like when, before performances, I joined hands and hearts with my costumed contemporaries in preparation for sharing our play with one another and willing audiences. I realize that there's an interdependent higher purpose to everything we say or do as individuals. Because beyond our outward shows of gender, age, ability, faith, or race, there is simply "us," players on the stage of life reuniting one play, one practice at a time.

The comedies, tragedies, and romances written (possibly) by an uncommon commoner from Stratford-upon-Avon highlight our shared humanity in profound ways. They encourage us to relax into the illusion of our dramas and mortal coils and to simply see them for what they are: a play unfolding. Dream-like, imagined bits of story that will one day melt into thin air. We get a sense of this metaphysical state when we are immersed in a well-staged Shakespeare play—or perform in one—and a sense of why I gravitated to yoga like iron to a magnet. Both Shakespeare and yoga are enduring reminders that when "the slings and arrows of outrageous fortune" (*Hamlet* 3.1) strike—and that, they do—we have provocative and mindful choices that relieve our suffering and give peace a chance; that right action matters. Our slowly evolving collective consciousness moves us toward the ultimate freedom.

Shakespeare's yoga shows us that consciously choosing to step into the spotlight of our shared inner light is a performance we can all participate in. And that applause you hear? That's the heavenly music of love, playing on, and on.

Bibliography

Adele, Deborah. *The Yamas & Niyamas: Exploring Yoga's Ethical Practice*. Duluth, Minnesota: On-Word Bound Books, 2009.

Bates, Laura. *Shakespeare Saved My Life: Ten Years in Solitary Confinement With the Bard*. Naperville, Illinois: Sourcebooks, 2013.

Bharati, Swami Jnaneshvara. "Yoga Sutras of Patanjali 1.1-1.4: What is Yoga?" *SwamiJ.com*. Accessed March 26, 2016. http://www.swamij.com/yoga-sutras-10104.htm

Bodhipaksa. "Krishnamurti: "It is no measure of health to be well adjusted to a profoundly sick society." Wildmind Buddhist Meditation. Last modified December 28, 2007. http://www.wildmind.org/blogs/quote-of-the-month/krishnamurti-measure-of-health

Carse, James P. *Finite and Infinite Games, A Vision of Life as Play and Possibility*. New York: Free Press, 1986.

Cope, Steven. *Yoga and the Quest for the True Self*. New York: Bantam Books, 1999.

Doris Duke Performing Artist Awards. "Shawn Sides." 2015. http://ddpaa.org/artist/shawn-sides/

Fahey, Caitlin Jeanne. "Altogether Governed by Humours: The Four Ancient Temperaments in Shakespeare." Graduate Theses and Dissertations. *Scholar Commons, University of South Florida*, 2008. http://scholarcommons.usf.edu/cgi/viewcontent.cgi?article=1229&context=etd

Farhi, Donna. *The Breathing Book: Good Health and Vitality Through Essential Breath Work*. New York: Holt Paperbacks, 1996.

Garber, Marjorie. *Shakespeare After All*. New York: Anchor Books, 2004.

Garber, Marjorie. *Shakespeare and Modern Culture*. New York: Anchor Books, 2008.

Greer, Germaine. *Shakespeare's Wife*. New York: Harper Perennial, 2009.

His Holiness the Dalai Lama and Howard C Cutler. *The Art of Happiness in a Troubled World*. London: Hodder & Stoughton, 2009.

Hosseini, Khaled. *The Kite Runner*. New York: Riverhead Books, 2003.

Hulse, S. Clark. "*Wresting the Alphabet: Oratory and Action in "Titus Andronicus".*" Wayne State University Press, *Criticism* 21, no. 2 (1979): need page numbers if applicable.

Iyengar, B. K. S. *Light on the Yoga Sutras of Patanjali*. London: Thorsons, 1993.

Iyengar, B.K.S. *Light on Life: The Yoga Journey to Wholeness, Inner Peace, and Ultimate Freedom*. Emmaus, Pennsylvania: Rodale, 2005.

Kripalani, Ed. K. *All Men Are Brothers: Life and Thoughts of Mahatma Gandhi as Told in His Own Words*. Paris: UNESCO, 1969.

Lennon, John. *Imagine*. Song. Ascot, Berkshire: Ascot Sound Studios, 1971.

Mabillard, Amanda. "Shakespeare's Longest Play." *Shakespeare Online*. Last modified September 20, 2004. http://www.shakespeare-online.com/faq/shakespearelongestp.html

Mathews, Amey. "Future Suffering Can And Should be Avoided, Sutra 2.16." *Yoga with Amey Mathews*. Last modified 25 July 2006. http://www.yogawithamey.com/futuresuffering.html

McKenna, Jed. *Spiritual Enlightenment, The Damnedest Thing*. Iowa City: Wisefool Press, 2002.

Morris, Sylvia. "Sadness and the Four Humours in Shakespeare." *The Shakespeare Blog*. February 18, 2004. http://theshakespeareblog. com/2014/02/sadness-and-the-four-humours-in-shakespeare/

Myss, Caroline. *Anatomy of the Spirit: The Seven Stages of Power and Healing*. New York: Three Rivers Press, 1996.

Newman, Allen. "Romeo & Juliet BroadwayHD Promo Clip (Orlando Bloom)." *YouTube* video. 4:51. February 3, 2014. https:// www.youtube.com/watch?v=HWPy584__gM

Patanjali. *Core of the Yoga Sutras: The Definitive Guide to the Philosophy of Yoga*. Translated by B.K.S. Iyengar. London: HarperThorsons, 2012.

Patanjali. *The Secret Power of Yoga: A Woman's Guide to the Heart and Spirit of the Yoga Sutras*. Translated by Nischala Joy Devi. New York: Three Rivers Press, 2007.

Patanjali. *The Yoga-Sutra of Patanjali: A New Translation with Commentary*. Translated by Chip Hartranft. Boston & London: Shambhala, 2003.

Patanjali. *The Yoga Sutras of Patanjali: A New Edition, Translation, and Commentary*. Translated by Edwin F. Bryant. New York: North Point Press, 2009.

Patanjali. *The Yoga Sutras of Patanjali*. Translated by Sri Swami Satchidananda. Buckingham, Virginia: Integral Yoga Publications, 2012.

Ram, Bhava. *The 8 Limbs of Yoga, Pathway to Liberation*. Coronado, California: Deep Yoga, 2009.

Renard, Gary. *The Disappearance of the Universe, Straight Talk about Illusions, Past Lives, Religion, Sex, Politics, and the Miracles of Forgiveness.* Carlsbad, California: Hay House, 2004.

Rumi, Jalal al-Din. *The Essential Rumi.* Translated by Coleman Barks. San Francisco, California: HarperOne, 2004.

Shakespeare, William. *King Henry IV, Part 1.* Introduction by David Scott Kastan. London: Thomson Learning, 2002.

Shakespeare, William. *The Riverside Shakespeare.* Edited by G. Blakemore Evans. Boston: Houghton Miller, 1974.

Showkeir, Maren and Jamie Showkeir. *Yoga Wisdom at Work, Finding Sanity Off the Mat and on the* Job. San Francisco: Berrett-Koehler Publishers, 2013.

Singer, Michael. *The Untethered Soul, The Journey Beyond Yourself.* Oakland, California: New Harbinger Publications, 2007.

Smith, Christian and Hilary Davidson. *The Paradox of Generosity: Giving We Receive, Grasping We Lose.* Oxford University Press, 2014.

Szabo-Cassella, Claire. "Muscular Dystrophy as a Source of Strength." *Australian Yoga Life* 41 (2014): 14 – 18.

Szabo-Cassella, Claire. "Shakespeare on the Mat." *Australian Yoga Life* 44 (2014): 12 – 17.

Thakar, Vimala. *Glimpses of Raja Yoga: An Introduction to Patanjali's Yoga Sutras.* Berkeley, California: Rodmell Press, 2005.

Wapnick, Kenneth. *Life, Death, and Love: Shakespeare's Great Tragedies and A Course in Miracles.* Temecula, California: Foundation for A Course in Miracles, 2004.

Films

Hamlet. Directed by Michael Almereyda. USA: Double A Films, 2000. DVD.

Hamlet. Directed by Gregory Doran. UK: BBC Wales, 2009. TV Movie.

Henry IV, Part 1. Directed by Dominic Dromgoole. London: Shakespeare's Globe Production, 2010. DVD.

Henry IV, Part 2. Directed by Dominic Dromgoole. London: Shakespeare's Globe Production, 2010. DVD.

Inequality for All. Directed by Jacob Kornbluth. USA: 72 Productions, 2013. DVD.

Inside Job. Directed by Charles Ferguson. USA: Sony Pictures Classics, 2010. DVD.

Macbeth. Directed by Eve Best. London: Shakespeare's Globe Production, 2013. DVD.

Much Ado About Nothing. Directed by Joss Whedon. Los Angeles: Bellweather Pictures, 2013. DVD.

Much Ado About Nothing. Directed by Kenneth Branagh. USA: Renaissance Films, 1993. DVD.

Much Ado About Nothing. Directed by Jeremy Herrin. London: Shakespeare's Globe Production, 2011. DVD.

Othello. Directed by Oliver Parker. USA: Castle Rock Entertainment, 1995. DVD.

Playing Shakespeare with the Royal Shakespeare Company. Directed by John Carlaw and Peter Walker. London: London Weekend Television, 1982. TV Mini-Series.

Romeo and Juliet. Directed by Don Roy King. USA: Broadway HD, 2014. DVD.

Romeo and Juliet. Directed by Franco Zeffirelli. UK: BHE Films,1968. DVD.

Shakespeare Behind Bars. Directed by Hank Rogerson. Kentucky: Philomath Films, 2005. DVD.

Shakespeare High. Directed by Alex Rotaru. New York: Cinema Guild, 2012. DVD.

Shakespeare Retold, A Midsummer Night's Dream. Directed by Ed Fraiman. London: BBC, 2005. DVD.

Shakespeare: The King's Man. Directed by Steven Clarke. Great Britain: Green Bay Media, 2012. TV Mini-Series.

Shakespeare Uncovered: Macbeth with Ethan Hawke. Directed by Nicola Stockley. London: Blakeway Productions, 2012. DVD.

Shakespeare Uncovered: The Comedies: Twelfth Night and As You Like It with Joely Richardson. Directed by Janice Sutherland. London: Blakeway Productions, 2012. DVD.

The Big Short. Directed by Adam McKay. USA: Plan B Entertainment, 2015. DVD.

The Way. Directed by Emilio Estevez. Spain: Filmax Entertainment, 2010. DVD.

The Wolf of Wall Street. Directed by Martin Scorsese. USA: Paramount Pictures, 2013. DVD.

Timon of Athens. Directed by Sebastian Kautz. London: Shakespeare's Globe Production, 2012. DVD.

Tracks. Directed by John Curran. Great Britain: See-Saw Films, 2013. DVD.

Wild. Directed by Jean-Marc Vallee. USA: Fox Searchlight Pictures, 2014. DVD

Index

About the Author

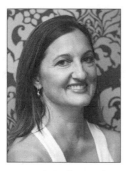 CLAIRE SZABO-CASSELLA is the founding codirector of Hot Yoga of New Zealand and its teacher training program. She contributes diverse articles on yoga to a variety of publications, including *Australian Yoga Life* magazine. She fell in love with Shakespeare's plays during her three summers (1985-1987) at Shakespeare at Winedale (Texas). She lives in Portland, OR.

Join the conversation about *Shakespeare's Yoga* on Facebook. Go to: https://www.facebook.com/shakespearesyoga/.